Rejuvenate Your Life

Rejuvenate Your Life

for mature women who want more in their *'Seenager'* years

Victoria Sheridan

Rejuvenation Coach
Lifestyle and Business Coach

Be youthful, healthy and happy
with the income security you want for your future

the Secret Calm

Published by
The Secret Calm Ltd,
Kent, England UK

Disclaimer

Every effort has been made to ensure that the information in this book is accurate. The information contained in this book will be relevant to most people but may not be applicable in each individual case, so it is advised that professional medical advice is obtained for specific health matters.

Neither the publisher or the author, accept any legal responsibility or any personal injury or other damage or loss arising from the use of the information in this book.

A catalogue record of this book is available from the British Library

ISBN 978-1-5272-65806

Media Enquiry

Victoria is available for interviews via

TV, Radio,

Podcast, Video and other media,

as well as appearances as a Guest Expert

on pancls and at events.

You are very welcome to contact Victoria via email:
victora@victoriasheridancoach.com
or visit her website: www.victoriasheridancoach.com

Victoria is a leading Rejuvenation Coach and she offers her Positive Lifestyle strategies which include stress relief and relaxation techniques. Her Business Success strategies help older women overcome their many concerns around ageing and income. Overall, Victoria's coaching and mentoring helps mature women to rejuvenate themselves and improve the quality of their lives as they become *'Seenagers'*.

Contents

~ Begin Here ~

Dedication

This book is dedicated to my two lovely daughters who have made this book possible, not least because at one time or another they have each generously given me the use of their laptops.

Without their unending support, faith and encouragement all the distractions and obstacles would have deflated me to the point where I would have given up on this project.

Thank you Angela and Elishia for helping me to bring this book into the hands and lives of all the glorious women that find comfort and inspiration inside these pages.

Foreword

I consider it an honour and a privilege to be asked to contribute to such an important book, so I did not hesitate in saying, *"Yes." when* I was asked.

As a Wellbeing Mentor and Author, I specialise in supporting others to feel happier and healthier following a major life change, such as a loss. My first book was published in 2019 and since then, I have been featured on Arianna Huffington's *Thrive Global*, as well as Radio Kent and Radio Sussex.

I first met Victoria via business networking in 2017 and I was immediately drawn to Victoria's energy and her desire to share her knowledge and expertise without being 'salesy' and pushy.

Over a short period of time, we discovered we have a mutual passion for helping others to feel better about themselves and to follow their dreams. As we are both artists selling our work, we are creative women and we both believe that expressing ourselves with art and writing is an important aspect of selfcare.

I have known Victoria for a few years now and during that time I have come to admire and respect her loyalty, her professionalism and her empathy. Victoria's passion for what she does oozes out of her every pore. In fact, I wish I had met her earlier on in my life when I was at a crossroads in my mid-40's following a major life change.

Everyone needs a Victoria in their life. I honestly believe that my first book probably would not have materialized and I would not be doing what I do now if I had not met her. She continues to be a trusted business confidante as I have a deep respect for her authenticity, honesty, and integrity.

Enjoy Victoria's wonderful book. Her zest for life is infectious and I guarantee you will feel inspired and empowered by her words and her vast experience as you transition into the next exciting phase of your life.

Wendy Jennings – The Coddiwomple Lady, Author of *From Cancer to Coddiwomple – A Story of Love and Daring to Dream.*
www.thecoddiwomplelady.com

Gratitude

To all my clients, I am grateful for the opportunity to work with you all over the years. You have inspired me with your courage and openness to rediscover and rejuvenate yourselves and your lives. You have attended my events in person and online and have fully immersed yourselves into my coaching programmes. I have learned so much from you and it is because of all your successes that I have now shared so much in this book with new readers.

I appreciate everyone featured in this book and those of you who have kindly expressed your feelings about being coached and having participated in sessions and events with me. I thank you all for sharing and celebrating your successes with readers through your testimonials, anecdotes and stories: especially, Sarah Corbett, Suzette McDowell, Denise Withey, Sara Squires, Cath Mills, Ann Williams and Jennifer Connelly.

To all the Guest Contributors who have written and shared chapters on your relevant and helpful specialisms, I appreciate all your effort and interest in bringing this book forward: Sarah Grant, Alison Wright and Julie Bartlett.

I also send a huge thank you to Author, Artist and Wellbeing Mentor Wendy Jennings for writing such a delightful Foreword and for all your support in so many ways.

What Others Say

"I had been struggling with ongoing stress and feelings of overwhelm, due to family problems but by the end of the sessions with Victoria, I felt so much calmer and happier. She taught me subtle techniques that worked immediately. Victoria has explained things to me in a clear way. I found it very helpful to learn how I can be in control."

Denise Whithey – *Health Centre Owner*

"Thank You Victoria. It was great that you listened to me and my needs and the sort of person I am. You made me feel confident about being as good as I can be, at everything that I do."

Sara Squires – *Early Years Education Trainer*

"Victoria's style instantly relaxed me while she helped me to break down some of my inner baggage. She shared with me some brilliant calming techniques to use discreetly and I would strongly recommend her. Thank you, Victoria".

Cath Mills – *Weight Management Consultant*

About This Book

Every woman from 45 years onwards should read this book. It speaks to all of them with issues about growing older, with concerns about their appearance, their vitality and their health and those who are worried about their financial security and especially about their relationships, being cared for and of course being happy.

What makes this book especially helpful is that Victoria shows mature women exactly, how they can move beyond the stress and challenges of any of the physical, mental and emotional transitions they experience at this stage of their lives and beyond.

She is very skilled at raising the hearts of women who feel disappointed or frustrated with the future they see themselves heading towards. Her coaching inspires self-belief and courage in older ladies who want the changes they are experiencing to be empowering.

Victoria is talented in helping women to rediscover who they are and unravel their sense of purpose. This is what enables them to reshape their health, their relationships and their finances so they can achieve the happiness they yearn for.

In these chapters, Victoria helps them rejuvenate their bodies, their feelings, their mindsets and their dreams. She has effective strategies and activities to show them exactly how to rediscover their *'mojo'* and how to have satisfying lives.

Ladies in these next stages of their lives often come to Victoria when they have reached a critical turning point. They know that '*things need to change*' but they have difficulty managing their stress and their feelings of being overwhelmed. They need support to have the clarity they need in order to find their best steps forward.

In truth, Victoria believes the specific help that she gives here, supports ladies who have a deep desire to re-define themselves and create the fulfilment they long for.

She was inspired to write this book because she considers all the women in the world to be an undervalued resource and Victoria refers to them as precious diamonds, recognising the beautiful multifaceted nature of women's personalities, values, priorities and dreams no matter who they are and what they want for themselves.

Introduction

Have you been crying lately? Have you been pacing the floor awake all night? Does time pass slowly no matter what you are doing? Are there many symptoms that you feel are dragging you down that you just cannot cope with anymore?

Whatever your personal situation, it is the biggest most difficult thing in your life at this time and what you are feeling right now is very real for you. Your feelings are painful but valid.

I have experienced these things too but despite the many and varied reasons for feeling stressed and overwhelmed, there are ways to stop the pain and control worry and anxiety by learning new ways to change your physical, emotional and mental reactions to conditions.

You CAN do this because it is simple; however, it is not necessarily easy and as everything in life takes practise you need to make a decision to at least try everything I share with you.

In this book I show you exactly how you can be free from stress and feel healthy, calm and youthful. You can learn ways to be actively involved with your wellbeing and to be healthier with more vitality. In the chapters ahead, you will find helpful techniques to swap feelings of anxiety for feelings of calm stability in any stressful situation. You will discover the best ways to build resilience and how to practise mindfulness and meditation well and you will also learn ways to easily enjoy a healing sleep and wake up feeling refreshed, vibrant and positive, ready to enjoy your life.

Understanding what is important to you and working out your true values and beliefs, helps you to make sure each of them is relevant and serves you well. Once you are sure that you have this understanding you can be certain that you are living a meaningful life with a motivating sense of purpose that drives you forward.

You can also have lots of useful resources and if you want me to guide you I have coaching programmes too that are designed to help you rejuvenate yourself and your life.

I am so excited for you because I trust that you will enjoy this book and I know you can be so much happier and enthusiastic about your future.

~ Finding Truth ~

Meet the Author

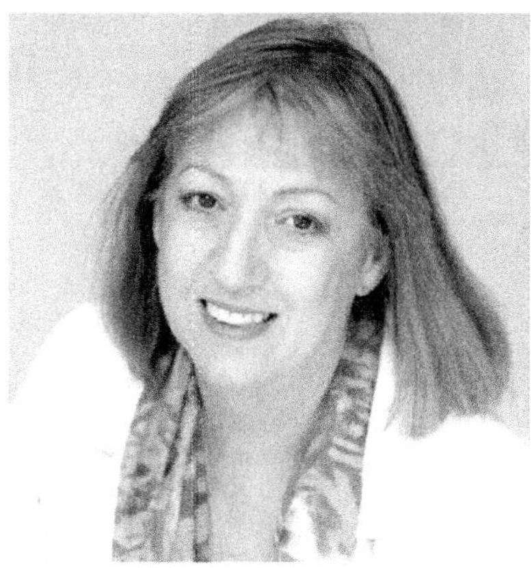

I am a fully qualified and successful Rejuvenation Coach and Business Coach to mature women and have worked with clients for over 30 years. During the early days of internet and FM radio I hosted my own life-coaching show in which I interviewed international celebrities and coached audiences via live phone-ins.

For many years I also enjoyed a rewarding career as a college and university lecturer in Kent and London.

Whilst building my career in education, I took on extra responsibilities and professionally coached many teachers, lecturers and students to improve their performance and achieve their professional goals. I love sharing my knowledge and expertise and I try to give more value than is expected of me in everything I do.

Alongside teaching I have also supported patients and health professionals in various hospices, dental practices, doctor's surgeries and charities. I share my own values through my work ethic and I value happiness and health and I also value relationships and making connections.

Throughout my varied experiences and opportunities, I have continually advocated for women to seek and find their personal happiness. I believe that all women can improve everything they do in life by finding their individual power and I love helping by providing platforms for them to express their own voices. Hence I help many of them to succeed in being self-employed or running their own businesses and to speak at relevant events and to write books.

.

****

All names of clients in the following chapters been changed for privacy and confidentiality purposes.

My Personal Passage

I took myself from *weary* to WONDERFUL

I finally gave up all the role playing and became a teenager again. Well, maybe not quite a teenager but it felt like it. I entered my 60's and I found I had turned into a 'Seenager'.

After being a responsible adult and raising a family as a lone parent, I also became a devoted grandmother. It was then, after having had a varied working life and a good career in education that like a teenager, I became resistant to the restrictions of my status quo lifestyle. I wanted to expand and have more freedom. Similar to when I was 18 years old, I wanted to explore what the world could offer me and find out what I could make of it.

For some time, my repeated the lament had been "*There has to be a better way to live*". Therefore, at 60 years old in my *'golden years'*, I found the courage I needed and I resigned from my job and my career. Fortunately, once I made that decision, I soon discovered that I was not the only woman who felt like that. In the months that followed, I met several other women who wanted the *'last phase'* of their lives to be more meaningful and satisfying. They joined me so they could learn how to become *'Seenagers'* too.

Once I had seized the day and grasped the opportunity to leave my career I was ready, willing and able to start my life over. Similar, to when I was an emergent teenager, I was very excited about my future but also reticent, not knowing how it would pan out. However, as an older and wiser *'Seenager'*, I sensed the world would open up to me and I had faith that it would give me new possibilities, different adventures and a chance to find greater joy and fulfilment.

Up to this point, I had already moved through several stages of life: from being a *protected* child, an *optimistic* teenager, a *supportive* wife and *nurturing* mother to my own children. I had also moved through the phase of being a career woman leading and supporting others through their academic successes to eventually transition into being a *devoted* grandmother and matriarch. Then, my career came to an uncomfortable end when I arrived at a point where I found I had changed. I looked and felt weary and I wondered what next? I had not quite realised it back then but I had entered the most significant stage of my life.

Amongst my colleagues and other peer groups I found many women who struggled with ageing and with the lifestyle and health issues they faced. I felt myself being drawn into the same negative thinking but it was making me unhappy. I resisted the expectation that I would grow old quietly and disappear into domesticity because since my youth, I had always believed that growing old would be a positive blessing and I would be of greater value to the world and the world would become even more interesting to me.

Eventually, I took everything I knew about modern scientific developments on ageing and the psychology around transformation. I considered all the different cultural values around feminine wisdom that I had studied throughout my life and soon I was no longer feeling lost.

As I reconnected with my authentic self and I clearly saw my own potential and how my future could be filled with purpose and motivation. I changed nothing about my family but I changed my life, regained my old dreams and formed fresh goals to suit me.

Once I had announced that I was in my *'Seenager'* years, I felt rejuvenated in so many ways. I was empowered and I moved forward, drawing on the experience and wisdom I had gained from already living a fascinating and interesting life. I realised I had become similar to my teenage self in that I had a wonderful opportunity to discover who I was and who I could be. However, more than that I wanted to shine and be vibrant and visible again. I refused to be a woman who settled quietly into in her *'autumn years'* and I quickly became a courageous *'Seenager'*. I decided to create a better life for myself and I wanted to be a voice to inspire other women.

Where am I now? Today, I have rejuvenated myself and reclaimed my confidence and zest for life; I am, happier and healthier. I also look younger than my years which means I feel great and exude a more vibrant energy. I now have a *'mission'* and I am moving my life forward with a daily sense of adventure, learning through different challenges and always expecting the best outcome. My personal mantra, since my early teens has been *"Expect the unexpected and that only good can come to me"*. Which means that I am open to new and exciting opportunities and when I experience disappointments or tragedies, I anticipate that there will eventually be positive outcomes.

Today, I live every day enjoying my new lifestyle in which I choose how I prioritise my work, my family, my health and my self-care and I am especially grateful for my daily *'me time'*.

Take yourself from *weary* **to WONDERFUL**

"Talk to yourself like you would to someone you love."

Brené Brown

Professor, Lecturer, Author and Podcast Host

My Professional Path

I went from *anxious* to AMAZING

Suddenly, my professional reset was underway. For several months I had planned to resign and kept the letter on my computer ready for the most appropriate opportunity. My 60th birthday fell in mid-April and the academic year ended at the end of June, so I submitted my resignation letter and my leave date was agreed. Within weeks, just before the end of the final term, I retired from my teaching career and was unemployed, but I felt relieved and excited.

In the years prior to resigning, I did not eat well, I slept badly and was constantly tired. I was post-menopausal for about 8 years and at that stage I did not understand that I was still in perimenopause. My energy levels were at an all-time low and I felt much older than I wanted to feel. I noticed my face was ageing, I rarely smiled, my hair was thinning and my dress code was dark and drab. My body felt heavy, I worried about my health and of course I lost my confidence.

When I entered teaching and became a lecturer, it was a vocation and it was important to me to *'make a difference'*; however, things had changed. My ideas were no longer given any attention and others talked over me which meant I no longer felt valued. I realised it was time for me to retire from what had become an exhilarating but exhausting career.

At first, I considered other employment but I was deflated, tired and confused. It was difficult to make clear decisions. I did not have the energy to undergo interviews for other jobs and promote my skills and *'sell'* myself to a new employer. I certainly could not face more studying or training and quite honestly, the thought of starting over at the age of 60 seemed too daunting.

However, a great yearning had risen in me, urging me to grow and do something significant with the next phase of my life. I had reached all the professional goals that I originally set myself but quite sadly I eventually felt uncomfortable, unchallenged and increasingly unwilling to work the long hours expected of me. My loss of family time and poor quality of lifestyle as well as lack of self-care was my motivation to step away and leave my routine, my colleagues and my financial security. It was time to begin over again and as I approached this great reset I was not in a good place.

However, I made the decision and my resignation letter had been submitted. Suddenly, I felt amazingly free and optimistic about my future and I was happy and ready to redefine myself.

It was important to me to have an easier work life that still enabled me to help others and still *'make that difference'* but in a way that suited my own physical and emotional wellbeing, as well as my personal beliefs and values.

Years previously, I had experienced coaching with Anthony Robbins and a few other well-known coaches and I was so pleased with the results that I qualified as a coach myself. Within my teaching role I also qualified twice as a coach and so with 3 separate coaching qualifications, I started my first coaching business alongside lecturing. I loved the success of the strategies I applied and I went on to enjoy an interesting time hosting my own life-coaching show on a pioneering internet and FM radio station. During this time, I interviewed a number of international musicians, singers, authors, TV and film actors and comedians. The show also included 10 minute coaching sessions with live audience phone-ins and so you can imagine that at times it was wonderfully stimulating.

During my teaching career I worked extensively with students who experienced various forms of disability. I was often involved in stress relief programmes for students as well as staff and me also, took on extra roles coaching other members of staff to manage their performance and career choices.

Throughout my adult life, I had also volunteered as a relaxation and meditation practitioner helping patients and health professionals in hospices, dental practices, doctor's surgeries and charities to understand and relieve their stress and anxiety. Over the years, I had taught thousands of people to relax and meditate effectively. This had always been an extremely satisfying way to give back to society and was often life changing for many of my clients and students.

Therefore, it felt natural for me to combine my therapeutic experience, my professional stress management and my coaching skills to establish myself as a professional coach. It also made sense for me to use the connections I had made, along with the skills and insights I had learned to start up and run my own business. Since that decisive point, I have enjoyed every minute of being my own boss.

What do I do now? These days I focus on the wellbeing of other mature ladies and I feel passionate about my work them they also need to feel happy. I help these amazing women to overcome restrictions and limitations so they can redefine their physical, their emotional and their mental selves. They become visibly more youthful and they feel replenished, revitalised and rejuvenated.

In the process, they revisit the vision and enthusiasm they once had when they were younger and they combine these with the wisdom and experience they have now they are older.

I simply love helping other ladies to find their freedom and pleasure and learn to value their age and their wisdom. I encourage them to make the best of their appearance, to give the best of their skills and knowledge and to be proud of themselves whilst they embrace their dreams. The delight they feel when they decide what will fulfil them and what they want next is a delight to be part of.

My coaching programmes help women from all backgrounds and cultures as I bring together, current scientific knowledge with relevant ancient techniques, to produce a successful modern practice. Bio-hacking health and ageing with the most recent developments in Nutrigenomics, Neuroscience, Psychology and NLP is exciting. This means I tailor my programmes to their individual needs.

I now spend my days, happy and stimulated by fresh challenges and I am grateful that I spend half of my time content and relaxed and the other half inspired and excited by my mission to empower mature women so that they enjoy life and have the health, income and happiness they want.

Take yourself from *anxious* to AMAZING

This is for All Women

This book is to help all women realise their true value and how much the world needs them to be well in all aspects of themselves and their lives.

I believe the compassion, wisdom and spirit of mature women are more relevant and more needed than ever, in these times when better health and longevity have given us the opportunity to forge ahead *en masse* and to participate in local and global affairs in ways never seen before.

In order to bring the world into greater harmony, we all need to address our long-held issues around self-worth, self-esteem and self-empowerment. Therefore, as an older woman, mature with a deep sense of purpose, my aim is to raise the hopes, dreams and desires of my *'sisters'* who do not yet recognise their own beauty, creativity and significance or who have not yet discovered their path to happiness and self-fulfilment.

In this book I share exactly how I help women to be stress free, to feel and look youthful and to be proud of the way they present themselves. How they can be actively involved with their wellbeing and how they can be healthier with more vitality. How they can be paid what they are worth whilst they give the best of their skills and their wisdom and how to be creative and expressive and to be proud of themselves and their achievements.

Mature women do not need to become someone new or different, but they do need to return to their original potential because when they were born, each of them was already someone special.

Now, with greater life expectancy, they have more living to do and most still want to be kind and giving and share their wisdom. They still want to make a difference to other people's wellbeing and to inspire them, but these amazing women understand that they also need joy and freedom and they want to live the rest of their lives more on their own terms.

I wrote this book is to inspire all women to move forward positively with a daily sense of adventure, learning through their challenges and always expecting the best outcome.

I Saw My Future

The door to the village hall opened and in stepped a woman who furtively, made her way to the edge of the room, not wishing to be noticed. It took her some time to watch from the side until she picked her moment and walked across to me and sat down. It would have been easy to assume she was shy and cautious, but it became apparent that she was far from quiet and timid.

Ann and her husband were in their 50's and they were considering their retirement plans and financial provision. Well into her menopause, Ann felt drained and was anxious about her future both at work and in her marriage. She explained to me many of the stressful circumstances she woke up to every morning and that she was ready to leave both job and husband but felt stuck because of financial insecurities.

Ann embarked on my *'Be Happy, Be Amazing'* rejuvenation and lifestyle programme and after just a few weeks of having coaching and using the stress relief techniques that she learned, she began to feel calmer and more stable. Ann was making sense of her problems and her underlying concerns. In a short time, with a calmer emotional state and more stable mind-set, Ann could make some clearer decisions and so she set aside time to speak honestly with her husband.

Using The Secret Calm techniques, she found the most useful, Ann prepared herself in advance. When they sat together Ann spoke in a kind manner with a hopeful approach, she focused on a positive outcome for both of them and afterwards she said the experience was successful and *'heart-warming'* for both of them.

Ann came to realise that her unhappiness was more easily remedied than she had realised. She had been focused on the behaviours of everyone around her instead of trying to understand her own menopause and unrealistic fears around all of her relationships. She learned to accept some aspects and took action on other parts.

Together Ann and her husband reaffirmed their love and their commitment to each other and they took time to reassess their values and mutual goals for their life together as a close, loving couple. They jointly, decided to relocate their jobs and their home to Devon and despite Ann's negativity, they each secured new employment. They put their house on the market and even though, Ann doubted they would achieve a quick or smooth sale, their house was sold within three days and contracts were easily completed several weeks later. Everything was flowing for them much more smoothly than Ann had expected. She realised the blocks to her happiness had been in her own thinking and approach. Quickly and without hesitation, they found interim rental accommodation and started their new jobs.

When I spoke to Ann several months later, she was happy and in the process of buying a permanent home. Ann was happier than she had been for many years and she had lost weight, because of a slightly more active lifestyle. She was much calmer and eating and sleeping better and she was still using some of the techniques I showed her. She sent me a photograph and I saw straight away that she looked younger with a beautiful broad smile and a tiny twinkle in her eyes that I had not seen before.

She spoke enthusiastically about our coaching sessions and the techniques she had learned that were still helping her. Ann told me that not only was she grateful for my guidance but her husband passed on his thanks to me too. This was an extra bonus for me because even though I know my work is effective it was still lovely and encouraging for me to hear details of her success and happiness.

Ann told me she felt younger, more attractive and enthusiastic about life. She liked her job and financial affairs had worked out well. Ann laughed a little at the thought of how badly her life could have gone if she had not attended my class that evening. I suggested that it was her own readiness to take decisive action and her willingness to practise what I showed her that resulted in her quick transformation.

Ann emphasised to me that the tools I had given her to understand and manage her stress, were the key to her complete rejuvenation and her ongoing appreciation of her life. She valued our coaching sessions and the insights and refreshed energy she had gained and Ann knew she could continue to improve her life.

Eventually, we both shared our surprise at how quickly from our initial meeting in my meditation group, that Ann had stopped feeling stressed, her anxiety disappeared, her marriage, home and income was transformed. It was then, that I realised how much Ann had helped me too.

"Oh Wow!" I exclaimed as I put the phone down and everything suddenly clicked into place in my mind. It was literally, a *'lightbulb moment'* and my mind lit up as I fully understood what had happened. In that flash of insight, I saw exactly what process I had used and I understood how I had taken Ann through it so quickly.

Amazed and excited, I saw my own future clearly and I knew that I could help other women to experience similar rejuvenations. Not only could I help them find their happiness but I had also found my passion, my purpose and my own happiness. Overcome with a wonderful sense of joy, I felt inspired, full of life and ready to take action. I had rejuvenated Ann but Ann had rejuvenated me too. It was then that I began to redesign my future.

Since then, I have been running my own coaching business for several years and Ann has kindly referred a colleague to my Rejuvenate Your Life programme. I am always grateful for opportunities to help even more women; therefore, I have captured the essence of my practice here in this book for you. Now, I can show you how you can also be inspired to rejuvenate yourself, your health and your wealth because I truly believe you deserve to be and can be happy.

"Your 40s are good.
Your 50s are great.
Your 60s are fab.
And 70 is ******* *awesome!"*

Dame Helen Mirren
Actress and TV Presenter

~ Successful Ageing ~

Stress Less, Be Happier

Feeling Stressed Affects Everything

Being in a state of stress affects your physical health, your vitality and your mental and emotional wellbeing. It affects your relationships, your work and productivity as well as your financial decisions and of course, worry and anxiety makes you look and feel older than you need to.

Also, although stress feels terrible, it can motivate you to avoid the source of your pain and discomfort and it is often the driving force that compels you to make changes in one or all areas of your life.

However, the quality of your life and your ability to look young and feel young with the hope and expectation of good health as you age, largely depends upon your ability to adapt to circumstances and your ability to be resilient and maintain an optimistic outlook.

These next pages help you to understand yourself before you focus on building your resilience. Then if you wish to you can find the courage and strength to transform yourself and your life.

Be aware that you may be going through changes but that these also effect other people around you. It can be in your best interests to understand why they may behave and react to you in negative ways and it can be helpful to know the reasons why you may not be getting the support you need and want from them. Difficult situations can be made much easier when you understand why the people who love you, try to hold you back from making the positive changes you long for. Keep their struggles in mind as you continue through the chapters ahead because those that are close to you can become your strongest allies during times of change and you may need them.

Stress is a signal that you feel threatened so your brain quickly becomes super focused with heightened intensity, on that threat and it rapidly searches for your best solution. However, in general, constant fear of imminent attack or death is unlikely and most daily stress is usually caused by complications in normal situations and relationships. This means that having an intense response to stress, is unnecessary but your brain responds with alarm and your thinking becomes confused which in turn, causes more stress.

This means you are unable to hold on to thoughts and ideas because they seem to either flow into each other or disappear into vagueness. When this happens, you continue to spiral into worry and overthinking things. However, all this worry can be futile and exhausting for you.

The solution is not as simple as killing a raging bear or running away. Searching for solutions, being in a state of high alert means that feeling stressed frequently leads to you feel confused and unable to focus. It feels as if you cannot control this internal dialogue or the internal current of emotional churning. This causes even more stress and the cycle of feeling vulnerable and anxious continues.

The fear of further anxiety can bring on panic attacks and other serious symptoms, so it is important to react to life as calmly as possible. Resilience is the key to being balanced and in control but can only be achieved when you repeatedly practise changing your current physical, emotional and mental states on a moment by moment basis.

What is Stress?

The first thing you need to know for sure, is that stress damages your cells. They literally die off because stress sets off chemical and hormonal reactions in your body that accelerate the ageing process. When you are young, your body's inbuilt recovery systems include tiny mitochondria in your cells that replenish and restore each one.

Unfortunately, as you age this ability for cellular repair decreases and you have fewer healthy cells.

How you respond to stress shows in your outer appearance, your skin, hair, eyes to lack lustre and triggers your internal structure and stamina to decline. Limiting cellular stress keeps your cells healthy and revitalised which helps you to maintain and regain your youthful looks and vitality. Having a rejuvenated body and a stress free, healthier and happier future depends on how you respond to stress.

Feeling fearful and overwhelmed is your reaction to a particular situation or set of circumstances that you believe are a threat to you in some way and your response is a quick reflex to save you from an urgent and harmful situation.

This is normal and a regular part of being human and is intended to arouse your survival instinct and avoid danger when needed. At the same time, it can be beneficial to your wellbeing because it is your '*stress response*' that alerts you to opportunities and creative ways to tackle or escape threatening circumstances.

There is a saying, *'Necessity is the mother of invention'*. This means at times of stress and difficulty you have the ingenuity to find new solutions to old problems.

Over time, you have learned some helpful reactions that have been useful, therefore, you repeat them. These learned reactions can be so ingrained in you, that it feels normal and natural to react in these familiar ways. You assume your stress is in your personality. *"It's who I am. I can't change."* However, it is often learned behaviour and can be unlearned.

Being suddenly stressed when you are unprepared, such as in a traffic jam or being continually and consistently stressed such as in a highly demanding job, are both equally as damaging. Whether mild or strong, stress can be extremely uncomfortable, even painful and you may need help to stop feeling overwhelmed by worry and anxiety. You will find some powerful solutions to try in this book.

Stress Facts

- Stress happens when your environment gives you clues that make you aware of either a real or imagined threat.
- Stress is both biological and psychological.
- Stress involves your autonomic nervous system and your brain which release stress hormones into your bloodstream.
- Stress is your body's way of preparing you to physically survive the potentially dangerous or harmful situation by running or fighting.

All stress accelerates ageing. The key to looking and feeling young is to understand stress and to keep it to a minimum by building your resilience to tense and traumatic conditions. Learning ways to control how you respond to stress will help you to stay youthful.

5 F's

When you become fearful your immediate reaction is to stop and take a breath in, hold your breath ready to listen whilst at the same time you bend your legs ready to run. Then in an instant you choose the best response.

Do any or all of these apply to you?

Fight	I engage fully to deal with a situation.
Flight	I retreat from a situation to assess the threat.
Freeze	I feel stuck, unable to decide on any action.
Faint	I give up, it is too much for me so I deny the threat exists and opt-out of dealing with it, hoping it will go away.

Feint I *'play dead'* by pretending I am ill to buy myself time to wait for a new option to appear or for others to resolve it.

2 S's

There are 2 States of stress. Your experiences of stress depends on whether the root cause of your stress is brief and short-lived or drawn out and long-lived. You may experience both as one can lead into the other.

Have you experienced any of these?

Acute State

You feel threatened in a sudden or brief but straightforward situation. For example, unexpected disruption to normal life, receiving bad news, an accident, physical attack, medical diagnosis or operation, giving birth, job loss, personal disagreement, damage to your home, unexpected financial outlay or technology breakdown.

Chronic State

You feel threatened by a prolonged or ongoing and complex situation. For example, buying and selling a home, facing job loss or redundancy, long term study and taking exams, perimenopause and menopause, long term care of others, overwhelming debt, prison, divorce, uncertainty, domestic abuse, disability or illness.

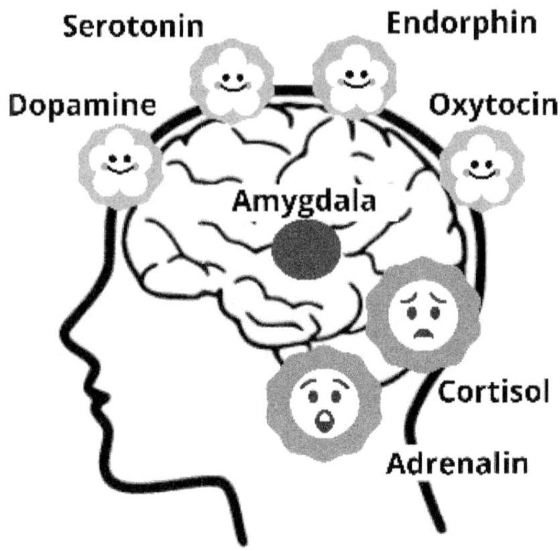

In simple terms, being in a state of stress involves chemicals and hormones. When your senses feedback to your brain that there is a possible threat then your amygdala rapidly sends messages via chemicals, to your body to make you ready for whatever might happen.

1. Amygdala receives the information about the threat.
2. Hypothalamus releases adrenalin and cortisol through your adrenal and pituitary glands into your blood stream.
3. This creates tension in your muscles, quicken your breathing and your heart rate.
4. Blood changes and flows from your major organs to your muscles.
5. You are ready to fight or run away.
6. Blood thickens in case you are injured.
7. Brain ignores any distractions.
8. You deal with or escape from the threat.

Your brain focuses on fight or flight and causes you to have difficulty thinking clearly and make wise decisions when you are feeling overwhelmed. In ordinary life it can make you worry and focus on the problem without finding a suitable solution. However, when you go over and over the same problem and think in circles, round and back again to the same thoughts, you then find it difficult to be calm. When you are fearful about a threat of any kind you soon blood stream is overwhelmed with these survival chemicals.

Once the threat is gone and the danger has passed, then your brain repairs your body and releases other chemicals and hormones to bring you into a safe state where you can relax and think clearly again.

These are *dopamine,* to make you feel satisfied and to relax your body; *serotonin* to make you feel sleepy and happy and to bring your body back to a normal state; *oxytocin,* to help you to feel safe as you can bond with your friends and family for support and endorphins which give you pain relief and a sense of euphoria.

If you have had a baby you may remember feeling these effects after childbirth. However, all of these chemicals and hormones are only designed to be released temporarily in an Acute State because during a long term Chronic State, these chemicals can cause harm to your body, your mood and your wellbeing.

Here are some common symptoms that can be caused by being overwhelmed.

Tick any of these which apply to you?

PHYSICAL

dizziness/palpitations
stomach cramps
nausea/vomiting
hyperventilating
lump in throat
panic attack
fatigue
constipation/diarrhoea
tingling fingers/hands
teeth grinding
loss of appetite
sudden weight loss/gain
menstrual changes
loss of libido
muscle tension /twitching/cramp
rocking/pacing
heart problems
high blood pressure
aches and pains
insomnia
sleep walk/talking
sleeping too much
handwringing
hair loss
low personal care
skin problems
gut acid/heartburn
nail biting
comfort eating

MENTAL

forgetful
vague
making mistakes
negativity
depression
obsessive
distracted
indecisive
worry
self-pity
anxiety
suspicious

EMOTIONAL

angry/lose control	mood swings
tearful/sad	overly sensitive
irritable	frustrated
lack of confidence	defensive

BEHAVIOUR

aggressive	workaholic
unrealistic goals	nervous
careless	late or absent
low social interaction	lying/deceitful
poor personal appearance	poor self-care
eating disorder	lethargy
poor personal relationships	addictions
rubbing/scratching	self-harm

General and Brief Descriptions

Severe mental health conditions need medical advice and support so see your doctor quickly to determine whether you need serious medical interventions.

Depression – *'fear of the known and remembered'*

Many scientists and medical researchers agree that a large part of feeling depressed involves dwelling on past events that cannot be changed. Depression can cause you to be stuck in a cycle of perpetual guilt, gloom, pessimism, confusion and powerlessness.

Anxiety – *'fear of the unknown and imagined'*

Professionals also agree that a prominent feature of being anxious involves dreading the future and anticipating the worst scenario of outcomes that could happen. Anxiety can cause you to be stuck in a cycle of perpetual worry, apprehension and nervousness as you struggle to find insight and solutions.

Both depression and anxiety involve deep feelings of unease, lack of clarity, confusion, fear, pessimism and hopelessness and it is possible to have both experiences at the same time by swinging between the two conditions. Where these overlap it is difficult to separate them and they often merge into one painfully muddled experience.

These symptoms can develop into chronic long-term conditions that affect not just your mindset and emotions but also your physical health and can also dramatically affect the way you age.

Short term and long term stressful situations can cause depression and anxiety and you can deal with these conditions by either avoiding the sources of the stress or if not, then by changing the way you react to them.

Medical intervention can be useful in intermediate to extreme cases however, in mild and moderate cases, a specialist coach or therapist may be worth considering. In this situation, you can benefit from a talking therapy working through your problems with a professional.

Chronic and acute stress can lead to low self-esteem and a continuous stream of inner dialogue with yourself can keep you trapped in a mental and emotional state of being constantly feeling insecure. Sadly, all this stress often results in physical deterioration and early ageing.

Finding alternative and complimentary ways to deal with depression and anxiety caused by stress can help and support medical interventions and the following chapters look at ageing and how to improve your health and longevity, staying a youthful *'Seenager'* as you manage your symptoms and move forward into a more stable and happier life.

"The best thing you can do in your life, have stillness and silence, to begin to appreciate yourself and to feel you matter."

Delia Smith CBE
Cook, TV Presenter and Author

Un-Stress Yourself Secretly

Stop Stress Related Signs of Ageing

Premature ageing due to stress, has been covered; however, there are things you can do to counteract and alleviate ageing and stay younger longer. You can take immediate action to alleviate and avoid further damage from the effects of stress.

The techniques I share in the next few pages are just a few that can help you to relieve and eliminate your anxiety and worries. You can achieve far more by joining my in-depth coaching programmes and you are very welcome to join me on social media.

The following pages include useful information, tips and exercises to give you stress relief, manage your anxiety and build resilience.

Tips for Self Help

Menopausal symptoms of tension, irritability and anxiety can be eased with techniques such as the ones I am sharing with you next. Knowing exactly how stress causes premature ageing is empowering because you can then take quick action to avoid and relieve its effects. You can do these exercises before and after any difficult situation.

The Secret Calm of *Comfort*

Tip 1 – Natural Relief

Whenever you are feeling overwhelmed, you can take control of your mood and make yourself feel safer, relaxed and happier. You can do this quickly by simply bringing your hands together and putting pressure into each palm.

Your brain senses from your body that you are being held and that you feel safe, relaxed, comforted and calm. Your body then responds by sending you into a deeper relaxed state. This is all very natural, simple and effective.

The technique I am explaining to you next sounds complicated but once you see how it looks and feels you will be fine, so try it.

Follow these directions before you begin the exercise.

Hold your relaxed hands side by side, face down in front of you. Your right hand is A and your left hand is B.

Turn B on its side. Move A across to B. Place the tip of your thumb from A into the palm of B. Let the fingers of A fold gently over the fingers of B. Relax. Place the tip of your pointing and ring finger of B into the palm of A.

Relax your hands. Gently press with a little force, into both of your palms at the same time. Your thumb is in one palm and 2 of your fingers are in the other palm. It is important to relax all your fingers.

You are holding your own hand with fingers pressing in one palm and thumb pressing in the other.

Tip 1 – Do This Now

Keep your hands gently folded over each other and press into your palms counting to 4 and then stop pressing and count to 4 again. Do this again counting to 8 and then stop pressing and count to 8. Lastly, press again and count to 10. Stop pressing and count to 10. Practise holding your hand in this way and counting whist you apply pressure to your palms.

Feel your shoulders drop as you being to feel peaceful.

Tip 1 – Science

Every baby is born pre-programmed to grab onto its mother and hold on for dear life, literally. You have probably experienced the strong grip a baby has as it refuses to let go of your hair. This is the *Palmar Grasp Reflex.* When anxiety kicks in you may try to replicate this by wringing your hands in an attempt to feel safe but a healthy alternative is to press gently but firmly into your palms. This triggers the release of dopamine and serotonin your *'happy hormones'*.

Even as an adult you seek the comfort of someone's hand when you are in pain and the feeling of being held is not just comforting, it is proven to ease your feelings of stress, anxiety, depression and insecurity. When you were an infant the sensation of your mother's body, the feeling of being held and especially when your mother held your hand gave you comfort.

Studies, show that women in particular need several hugs a day of at least 30 seconds to stay physically, emotionally and mentally well. When you hold hands in this way, your brain stops releasing stress hormones and floods your blood with calming and relaxing dopamine and serotonin to reinforce your feeling of being safe, cared for and looked after. This gives you feelings of trust that everything is going to be okay and fills you with peace and happiness.

This is a great result for you and is quickly achieved.

The Secret Calm of *Relief*

Tip 2 – Flowing Breath

Whenever you feel stress or worry, if you feel anxiety or pain, breathe in slowly to bring your heart rate down. This tricks your brain to reverse your stressful state, bring it back to normal and give you a happier and more peaceful mood.

You can do this quickly by simply breathing slowly and deeply. Breathe like a baby breathes when it sleeps. Let your tummy rise and fall by expanding and compressing your tummy instead of your upper chest. It is important to fill your lower diaphragm and not the top of your lungs. Practise a few times and relax into it.

Practise breathing in this specific way a few times and be patient. As you breathe in this way, your brain senses the motion. The motion informs your brain that you are already relaxed and feeling sleepy, so it stops releasing adrenalin and stress hormones.

This induces your brain to release more of the calming and relaxing dopamine and serotonin which make you feel safe and happy.

Tip 2 – Do This Now

Take a deep breath in and breathe out dropping your shoulders.

1 On a count of 4 breathe air in slowly. Imagine your tummy is like a balloon. Fill it up and extend it out.

2 Hold your breath, for a count of 4 with your tummy still extended and full.

3 On a count of 4 release your breath out slowly. Imagine the balloon emptying, deflate your tummy gently and relax.

Repeat, watching your tummy rise and fall just as it does when you are sleeping deeply and also, when you are feeling relaxed and calm. Breathe in slowly, breathe in deeply and breathe yourself well.

Tip 2 – Science

When you were born, your first breath was your initiation into the world. Since then, you have been sustaining yourself by freely taking from the abundance of air in the world around you.

Normally, when you inhale and exhale, the pressure of your breathing is balanced. However, when you are fearful and experience stress this balance is disrupted. Long term disruption and prolonged stress arouses your sympathetic nervous system and can cause it long term damage.

Studies show that slow deep breathing resets both the balance and the autonomic nervous system. Also, according to research, deep breathing involves the stress hormone cortisol and lesser-known hormones such as norepinephrine and epinephrine. These are proven to be regulated by deep breathing and this breathing exercise can improve the quality of your sleep.

When you hold your breath, your body has time to assimilate greater amounts of oxygen into your blood cells. This stream of enriched oxygenated blood reaches your brain and helps to regulate the release of your hormones.

Ultimately, by practicing this type of breathing from your lower diaphragm your body rises and falls, just as you did when you were a baby. This is your most natural way of breathing for sleep and deep relaxation.

When you initiate this breathing pattern yourself, you trick and convince your body and brain into believing you are already sleeping. Your brain then responds to your breathing activity by lowering the amount of cortisol and releasing more dopamine, endorphin and serotonin which you have already seen are your calming and '*happy hormones*'.

This gives you another quickly achieved result.

The Secret Calm of *Resilience*

Tip 3 – Visualisation

Resilience is when you can meet potentially stressful situations and circumstances without becoming stressed. However, if you do become stressed, then you can regain your balance and self-control quickly and stop yourself feeling stressed. You can do this by using specific techniques to maintain a constant state of calm and then you can give an appropriate response that serves you well and keeps you safe.

Visualisation is a natural process that I have been teaching for over 40 years and if you commit to practicing and learning this technique, then you can become resilient to stress and enjoy a happier life.

Tip 3 – Do This Now

Before you start read through **Tips 1 & 2 – Do This Now**
(If you prefer you can ask someone to read these instructions to you.)

Now, close your eyes and imagine you are opening your fridge.

You see a chilled apple inside.

Pick up the cold apple and feel it in your hand.

Now leave your home and imagine you are walking.

It is a pleasant walk and you look at gardens as you go by.

You arrive at the entrance to a park and walk in.

Imagine you are walking across the grass.

Find a sturdy tree and sit on the grass beside it.

Lean against the tree and feel a soft breeze on your face.

Look up at the blue sky and the bright sunshine.

Enjoy the scene and feel yourself smiling.

Slightly open your eyes hallway and keep them relaxed.

Repeat this affirmation slowly and out loud in a soft voice.

The Earth holds me – The Tree cradles me

The Sky soothes me – The Sun inspires me

Finish the exercise by smiling and then breathe normally.

Tip 3 – Science

In terms of psychology, researchers agree that anxiety is when you dread the future and anticipate the worst scenario and outcome.

In terms of biology, I previously showed how you react to threats by adapting your behaviour when your brain releases chemicals that stimulate your flight or fight responses.

Studies have shown that various forms of meditation and mindfulness have a beneficial effect and over time, with practise can build resilience to situations and conditions that make you feel overwhelmed and stressed.

In my programmes, I use *The Secret Calm* techniques to simply reverse this process by tricking your brain to release the opposite chemicals and hormones, so that you feel calm and relaxed, with an open mind ready to recognise solutions you need to feel safe. Breathing deeply, pressing your hands and imagining things that make you feel happy relaxes your body and sends messages to your brain that you feel comforted and safe so your brain releases dopamine, serotonin and stops releasing oxytocin and adrenalin. You feel refreshed and alert but deeply relaxed and calm, which improves your creativity and problem solving and as you saw previously, it helps your cells to renew themselves.

This gives you another quickly achieved result.

Meditation Is Key

Peace and Youthfulness

When you understand how your brain works you realise why it is important to persist at practicing meditation. It is not enough to try it once or twice and give up. Even if you experience difficulty, do not decide that you cannot meditate because this is highly unlikely.

I am going to use the analogy of an apple tree.

You know that many different people can reach up and pick an apple from a tree; children, short people, tall people, busy people, tired people and people who need assistance. They can all enjoy the apples.

However, when you go to pick apples sometimes the tree is full but other times the tree is empty or there is only blossom, or sometimes the apples are rotten, or the best ones are high up and out of reach. Sadly, you might not succeed in enjoying the full tasty experience of an apple precisely when you wish to and you may be disappointed.

The reason for this is some people have knowledge and experience whilst others do not. These people know there is a process the tree goes through, in order to produce the lovely juicy apples. They also know that although they may visit the tree and enjoy the beauty of the blossom but they understand that the apples are only ready to be picked at a certain stage of the process when they are fully grown and ripe. Therefore, they still visit the tree but they do not become upset if they do not find apples.

They have learned from their experiences when the best time and conditions are in place. Then when they visit the apple tree they find lots of delicious apples.

The secret to meditation is similar to the fruit on the apple tree. You need to recognise and accept the stages you need to go through to eventually experience the reward of a satisfying or wonderful meditation.

Practise the process and you can learn to gently move through the different stages of consciousness to reach the really happy state of deep meditation.

Remember there are many levels of relaxation and there are many reasons why meditating is good for you. It is very natural and far easier than it sounds. After all, children and people of all ages achieve the calm they need and so can you.

However, my point is that if you have difficulty meditating then you need to be patient and let the science work for you. Here are some examples of the levels you can expect to go through at different times and with various levels of success whilst you are learning.

A word of advice if you are in a group, never measure your own progress against what others tell you they experience. We all fluctuate and it is about working on your own resilience and your progress is your affair.

Return to meditate often, starting with a few minutes and then letting the time expand naturally. It is not a competition it is for you to be happy. Only be guided by your own joy and follow your own pleasure when you meditate.

Meditation and Brain Health

According to science, your body including your brain begins to deteriorate when you reach your early 20s. Since the availability of EEG and fMRI scans there have many studies into effects of meditation on the brain and ageing. However, there are both ongoing and fresh studies that continue to discover major surprises which have overturned our previous beliefs about your brain. Science now has evidence that meditation alters your brain matter as well as your brain and mind capacity. These results demonstrate that meditation encourages a healthy body and a positive mind.

According to eminent researcher Eileen Luders, from University of California, when you meditate there are micro and macro changes in your brain which increase the amount of grey matter and these can counteract the loss that occurs during the ageing process. This means that meditation can increase your brain health.

Meditation has also been shown to slow down or halt the progression of mild cognitive impairments such as the early onset of Alzheimer's disease. Meditation also protects your grey matter by reducing stress levels and at the same time reduces the harmful gene expression; as you saw earlier in chapters covering nutrigenomics, epigenomics and ageing.

Also, the results of other studies show that regular meditation helps you create healthier lifestyle habits especially around sleep, nutrition, work, movement and exercise. It also raises your self-awareness and raises your expectations and aspirations you have for yourself. Studies have shown that when you commit to meditating regularly, you increase your intelligence and increase your consumption of knowledge. You also, tend to increase your social and your financial status and wellbeing.

Most importantly, meditation is a popular way to relax and enjoy some inner quiet and peace. The psychological benefits, the mental and emotional benefits and the physical benefits are freely achievable by everyone who sits or lays down with the intention to breathe deeply and create a calm state. Being relaxed gives you brighter thoughts with which you can make clearer decisions and help you feel balanced and optimistic.

When you are finding your way through menopause, when you are looking for change or when you are creating change, meditation can give you everything you need to be successful in the world and in your heart.

If meditation is a step too far for you right now, then Mindfulness can make a difference to your mood, your mental and emotional health and give you more tools to improve your sense of wellbeing.

Actress Sheila Hancock says, *"What I try to do is not just say, "Isn't that bowl of flowers lovely " and go on. I try to dwell and I say to myself, "That is lovely and it is making me feel happy. ... Every now and then I say, " I am happy now with the sun on my back and lovely people around me."*

Taking time to stop and choosing to be present in that moment helps you to recognise the beauty in small things. This can give you pleasure and is calming. It gives you a space to think and sense clearly and to feel as Sheila says, 'happy'.

Age Well, Live Well

How to Build Resilience

Understanding how stress happens empowers you so that you can improve your resilience. Then, as you learn to control your reactions and stop responding to many of the triggers, you can delay signs of ageing within your cells, your body and also your brain.

Although, feeling stressed is a coping mechanism and you can appreciate it is necessary for your survival, there are also, many situations when you feel stressed, that are not life threatening. As you realise that much of the stress you feel is unnecessary you can build resilience by controlling your reaction to any threatening situations. You can practise powerful calming techniques that help you avoid feeling stressed and overwhelmed. Eventually, you can use your mental strength to stop yourself from feeling stressed before it occurs.

The key word is *'practise' and* it takes time and effort. This is why you may benefit from being coached until you master the skills you need to learn. Your next step is to decide which circumstances are real threats and which are only perceptions and you can continue to build your reliance and maintain a sensible attitude.

When you continually react to non-serious situations with fear you can be overwhelmed on a daily basis. This can mean you experience unhealthy levels of stress. Your worries compound over time until you eventually create a chronic state of fearfulness, apprehension with negative thinking and beliefs. This pessimism can make your life miserable and make you lethargic, apathetic and your behaviour is ageing giving the impression that you are much older than you are. Frown less and smile more to appear younger.

Some studies on the effects of stress show that anticipating and expecting situations to be stressful and then worrying and being anxious about them, is as harmful to you as actually being in them and living them. Yet, you may be one of the many women who believe worrying and being anxious is a good thing because you may believe you are preparing for the worst and you may even believe you are not a good and conscientious person, wife or mother if you are not worrying. Fortunately, most situations are unlikely to ever be as bad as you imagine them to be but unfortunately, your brain does not know the difference between real events and imagined events especially when strong emotions are involved. Your brain believes and acts upon everything you tell it and show it so, monitor and swap your negative thoughts quickly to positive ones that make you feel happier or at least more hopeful. Practise being hopeful.

Avoid Stress to Avoid Premature Ageing

Your resilience to stressful situations can increase your positivity and replenish your energy and sense of adventure in life. You can *'grow older and grow bolder'* but if you are prone to feeling stress often, then the amount you could tolerate and cope with when you were younger, decreases with time. When you were young you could quickly recover from the effects of stress; however, as you have already seen, being in chronic state of fearfulness, worry and stress is far more damaging and causes physical and mental deterioration. Worrying about getting older, putting on weight, being less attractive, having less money and disposable income, losing your focus in life and being fearful of the future, coupled with poor sleep can cause you to age quicker.

There is good news though and the following chapters help you to manage your stress, balance your emotions, improve your mindset and helps you to strengthen your body and your overall wellbeing. Your resilience and the de-stressing techniques shared here will not only enable you to achieve this but they will help you to look younger and have the cellular age of at least 10 years younger; plus, you will feel rejuvenated inside and outside.

With renewed vitality you have the confidence you need to be happier and you regain your clarity to make sound decisions for your future. Having the facts about how stress causes premature ageing is empowering because you can take clear action to avoid its effects.

Anti-Ageing

In many ways Anti-Ageing is about believing that the limitations of ageing can be overcome and that mindset and self-belief can defeat the ageing process. This approach is in favour of resisting growing older and celebrating youthfulness instead by investing effort, time and resources which are devoted to valuing and preserving youth and looking younger for longer.

Anti-Ageing means to continue to be active and to participate in adventure and endeavours. This modern era encourages you to be healthy and fit with high self-esteem and to engage with fully with life. This confident and optimistic approach encourages you to preserve your youthfulness by avoiding ill health in older age.

The Anti-Ageing approach often suggests that you should work throughout your life and sustain your strength and energy with a healthy lifestyle. This includes going to the gym often or taking regular exercise to maintain a body weight and physique that is now expected of you and inference suggests you should support yourself financially throughout your life.

However, I meet women who tell me that they are beginning to feel pressured into being someone they are not able to be anymore. It may be a great idea to be healthy and not accept a decrepit and old age in poverty as a given but, is everyone able to sustain the effort needed to be physically, mentally and emotionally perfect and also have an optimum level of health?

For example, I meet many 50 and 60 year old ladies who feel they are expected to follow fashion trends and to be sexually active when they would rather focus on other things. I also meet women who tell me they like to look attractive and well for their age but feel anxious about using beauty treatments and surgeries to give the illusion of being younger than they are. Nevertheless, they regard ageing as being unattractive and the search for youthful looks and energy is often motivated by the fear of missing out in life and not being accepted as they age and they feel this is putting pressure on them to have aesthetic treatments and surgeries.

This is because ageing can often mean a drop in income and many older mature women tell me that these pressures cause them to feel inadequate. They often find that gym and salon fees as well as keeping up with fashion becomes more difficult as their income diminishes. One of the things that concerns menopausal and postmenopausal women is resembling their mothers and looking older than they need to as well as losing their sex appeal, on top of losing their status, their success and their income. However, they also want to sleep more, relax more, mellow more and slow down yet they feel pressured to perform and be vibrant at times they do not want to. Very often they do not feel they can or should say, "No." to situations or to people and so they often feel torn between their own desires and pleasing others. They struggle to assert their own wishes.

Many mature women tell me that their own children will not allow them to be older or acknowledge they are changing. *"You're not old mum! Age is just a number"*. However, so many of my clients say that it does not help when their own family members do not acknowledge they have a right to feel older some days and its normal to want to stay indoors or maybe have a power nap or even a sleep in the afternoon.

I remember when I was in my mid 50's onwards, just after menopause and working full time, more like 24/7, that if I dozed on the sofa, someone in my family would soon wake me up and tell me I was too young to be napping yet. This was despite that I was catching up on all the times I could not sleep well at night. My family seemed to think I was *'giving in to old age'* too soon. Personally, I think they were simply afraid of facing the fact I was growing older. Once I retired and managed my own diary I slept better and also, the term *'retired'* enabled them to get more used to the idea of my ageing. I understand they wanted me to stay the mum they had always known but they did eventually learn to leave me to sleep if I nodded off.

Anti-ageing notions also mean you may have some resistance to growing older because you feel patronised by your family, especially by your own children. Women tell me they find it challenging to let go of being the parent and provider. They have difficulty to passing the decision making to their children as they cling on to their matriarchal roles and the responsibility they feel to still provide financial support for their children, They worry and feel guilty that as they grow older they may not be able to afford to maintain the financial support they are used to giving their children and they can experience loss of self-esteem because of this.

Lots of ladies also, resist appearing older when it comes to asking for help because they feel embarrassed and often feel insulted when help is offered. They have spent their lives looking after everyone so letting go of the role and the sense of empowerment they have in that role, is not easy for them; especially if they have not yet found a substitute or alternative role.

I found that I was not the only woman to deal with this, resistance to ageing as clients had similar stories. Even when they age a little or a lot, women are often denied the lifestyle changes and slower pace that they want and need.

There are positives and negatives regarding the Anti-Ageing approach to valuing youth and trying to reverse the ageing process. What inevitably happens though, is that women disapprove of themselves and can even hate their appearance so much so that they turn to many expensive products, invasive treatments and surgeries in order to achieve the illusion of youth. Therefore, mature women are often insecure and somewhat anxious about themselves, still unable to truly value and accept themselves.

Themes around lack of self-esteem and lack of confidence can often sadden them and undermine them even their later years especially once money becomes scarcer and they cannot afford the enhancements they want. This slow erosion of their finances is an aspect of women's wellbeing I like to help mature women focus on and I enjoy helping them to find other streams of income to support the lifestyles they want.

Pro-Ageing

Pro-Ageing is about loving age and enjoying the benefits of being older. It concentrates on women celebrating their age and looking forward to the later stages of life. Each age brings different challenges and rewards and more than wanting to look young again, most older women enjoy the pleasures of their mature, wiser years. Pro-Ageing promotes the idea of being true to your authentic self. Embracing your grey hair and wrinkles and appreciating the signs of a well lived life and the wisdom and experience that mature women bring to the world. This does not mean women should not use cosmetics or hair dye but they can also be just as attractive by enhancing their natural good looks and exude natural confidence if they choose not to. After all, smiling and being happy makes every woman beautiful.

Pro-Ageing is about valuing the contribution and the experience as well as the grace and the beauty of mature women. It promotes the beauty of ageing and welcomes the signs of ageing such as lines and greying hair as a natural development that women should accept and be proud of. Pro-Ageing is also about not following outmoded ideas about women becoming worn out but rather as valuable treasures that enrich our families and societies. Individually, women can also decide to redefine themselves and choose to love themselves. They can opt to live the healthiest lifestyle that suits them as they mature gracefully.

Fairy Tales

Why do older western ladies feel so badly about themselves that they feel they need to struggle with the ageing process? If we are surrounded with older women such as grandmothers when we are born and we feel their love and support why do we often as a society, fear being like them?

It can often be because of the influence of subtle conditioning and societal expectations that our role models have had a negative impact on us. Our grandmothers may have had their own negative issues about growing older and pass these feelings on to us; however, there are also other experiences when we are young children, that can reinforce our negative views of mature women.

For example, many western children of all genders, are brought up with negative examples and images of older women in the stories they hear and read in their very early years.

Think back to Little Red Riding Hood who takes responsibility for visiting her aged grandmother who is frail and weak, lives alone and is the reason the innocent young girl is placed in danger. This older woman may be sweet but she is portrayed as being a useless burden.

Quite often in fairy tales, the mother has died in childbirth or soon after and the child is left abandoned by her. Think about Snow White. The mature stepmother in this story is obsessed with her appearance and her lost youth and beauty. She is portrayed as a powerful queen with authority but is jealous of Snow White's highly valued beauty. This older woman is cunning as she deceives everyone into believing she is glamourous and beautiful. She becomes a dangerous woman committed to preserving the power she believes youth gives her.

Historically, because many women did not survive childbirth, it was common for stepmothers to step in and look after the child and family. Yet these helpful stepmothers are often depicted in these stories as cruel old hags, who use trickery and lies to get their selfish ways.

Although, there is a godmother in Cinderella and another in Sleeping Beauty, Godmothers are traditionally fairies who are not human and it takes supernatural intervention for them to help the innocent and vulnerable girl. The love and power of the Fairy godmothers comes from another world of magic and it can be said that they represent the loving spirit of the lost mother.

However, in all these stories, older women are always vilified and either made out to be a liability such as in Red Riding Hood, or a danger. They are portrayed as evil, which is the polar opposite of the kind, innocent young girls who are the exemplars of goodness. It is no surprise then, that women in western societies have a dread of growing old and why menopause is seen as a terrible ending rather than a doorway to a new beginning. Can you think of any fairy tales where an older man is depicted as being so evil because his age causes him to lose his looks and his power or because he steps up to look after step-children?

The Pro-Ageing approach suggests that women are beautiful just as they are; as nature intended, whether younger or older. This particular approach values ageing and attempts to change the deeply ingrained negative ideas, attitudes and beliefs about mature women. Being Pro-Ageing is about respecting mature ladies for their experience and wisdom and just as the lines on a man's face is seen as signs of experience and strength, so too can the lines on a woman's face, be seen as signs of feminine endurance and wisdom having lived a long life.

Mature women in their *'golden years'* are encouraged to enjoy their later years free from anxiety and self-loathing by developing high self-esteem with high levels of confidence. Pro-Ageing also sees mature women as excellent role models, for younger women as the wise intuitive healers and the educators of the next generations.

Mature Women in the Media

Media is generally, magazines, brochures and posters, films, theatre and events, radio and television broadcasts and the internet in all its platforms.

Being invisible in terms of the media has long been reinforcing the lack of self-worth that many older ladies feel and it can affect their mental and emotional health and well-being. Invisible Woman Syndrome (IWS) is a real thing and women are very aware that they are seen as being less relevant as they mature. Until recently, ageism was a big problem in Hollywood, TV and magazines and we have come a long way and achieved more roles and positions for mature female professionals largely because women have written the parts or become directors and producers themselves. Despite improvements though women are still fighting to remain in front of camera in TV and magazines which are still generally biased towards youth and beauty.

This also, remains a very difficult situation for career women in leadership roles in business, politics where a woman's age and relationship status are still mentioned in news items and features. In the workplace and corporate board rooms, women do not want to be replaced as it makes them feel displaced and disrespected, without value or purpose.

Yet it is perfectly natural in the scheme of life and after the transition there are many benefits and freedoms to be gained when you let go and pass the batons over to the next generation whether at home or at work. Mutual respect is the key to the successful handing over of responsibility and the sharing of wisdom and it is worth achieving this, if possible, to open up to a new lifestyle around your own needs instead.

What role does the media have in this reluctance by many women, to allow others to step up? In the past, mature women were rarely seen on the TV and film screens until they were old enough to play elderly grandmothers. Whilst their male counterparts could work throughout any age and stage of life, women could not deliver the news or present programmes past 40 years old and they could not even play the wives of older men because it was always an *'accepted norm'* that those men had much younger wives. Apparently, it helps the ratings when younger women are used but men are generally, still regarded as desirable when they have matured.

This has changed to some extent in recent years as women have blazed the trail to be directors, writers and producers and created more preferable roles for themselves. In TV and film, there is an increase in strong parts for mature women and research shows that there is a general belief that women are now being portrayed more positively in all the media.

However, this can be a misguided belief as current studies show that nearly all women's magazines in the UK, who despite having older readers, rarely use images of older women and if they do, they tend to only present celebrities who are happy to appear younger and sexier than they usually are and as we know, the use of air brushing and filters is common.

Images of older women are generally of mature models who have remained lean, fit and attractive and magazines still rarely use a wide variety of images of ordinary middle-aged ladies. You will usually find women younger, than the readers in these magazines because many editors and publishers still believe the flawed premise that older women prefer to look at images of women they aspire to be like. They assume older readers do not want to look at their own age group.

Such magazines seem to have an agenda that promotes age denial, because, like the cosmetic industry, they regard ageing as a problem that needs to be fixed where possible. The assumption by many editors is that ageing is unsightly to readers and therefore, not to be included; unless an eccentric aged model, designer or artist is included as an example of rebellion with a positive but *'edgy'* attitude to ageing that is to be celebrated; even though this is far from the experience of ordinary women. The result is that although the readers of these magazines are middle-aged, they do not find many images of women like themselves in them.

Generally, if magazines include an image of a mature lady, they use a small image and place it amongst a group of several other images. If a larger image is used the woman is usually within a group that contains other generations and in both scenarios, the focus is taken away from the more mature woman. Mature ladies are often lost or hidden amongst the multigenerational crowd whether in one image or several smaller ones.

It is not surprising that older women feel they are invisible.

"I'm baffled that anyone might not think women get more beautiful as they get older."

"Confidence comes with age and looking beautiful comes from the confidence someone has in themselves."

Kate Winslet CBE
Actress

Wear Your Genes Well

The Science of Ageing

For those of you who like to understand the science that underpins the many theories about ageing, you need to carry out your own investigations into what current research shows about ageing well. Meanwhile, in this chapter, I give you a summary of the main theories and ideas albeit basic.

When you think about your longevity you probably think of the end part or your life and the process of ageing in terms of physical degeneration and mental decline with loss of mobility, limited lifestyle and probably lack of dignity.

Yes, modern science is also interested in improving the quality of your health in those later years but the reality is that science is also interested in extending your younger, healthy and active years. I believe the longevity you want is not just an extended *'lifespan'*, but also a rejuvenated vitality and an extended '*healthspan'*.

I am just covering a few main theories here so that you can see how you can be more optimistic about your anticipated longevity. According to researchers who specialise in ageing, there are several theories about how humans age and some of these models work alongside each other to undermine our health, wellbeing and optimum youthfulness.

If you could look inside one of your cells, you would see that various parts of all cells communicate with each other via signals. As you grow older this communication becomes weakened and greatly reduced. In the next few pages, I will explain, in basic terms, some of the ways you can remedy or reverse the decay of your cells and delay your body's ageing process. You can do more in-depth research yourself to understand these processes more deeply.

Common Signs of Aging

Wrinkles	Grey Hair
Eyesight loss	Hearing Loss
Memory Loss	Confusion
Headaches	Muscle Pain
Noise Sensitivity	Slowness

Common Age-Related Illnesses

Infections	Asthma
Diabetes	Osteoporosis
High Blood Pressure	Stroke
Atherosclerosis	Fibromyalgia
Alzheimer's	Parkinson's
Chronic Fatigue Syndrome	Arthritis

Stay Youthful and Protect Your Health

When you are young your body produces enough natural antioxidants to regenerate your cells and maintain your vibrant health and youthfulness. However, after the age of about 20, your production of antioxidants decreases and your body begins to age.

Antioxidants are chemical reducing agents that protect your cells by removing electrons and hydrogen from them to keep them healthy and free from oxidation and deterioration. As your body's production of antioxidants dramatically decreases with age the protection against oxidation and disease weakens and oxidation of the cells causes them to die.

Therefore, to prevent and slow down, or in some ways reverse the degeneration of your cells, you need to avoid *'free radicals'* because they cause oxidation and decay.

To stay fit and healthy with youthful vitality and to look younger, you can introduce more antioxidants to destroy 'free radicals' in large quantities, through your diet and supplements. Consuming foods with high antioxidant value help you to stay fit and healthy with youthful vitality and to look younger for longer.

Avoid stressful situations because your stress response releases cortisol which increases your levels of oxidative stress which in turn triggers further stress responses. Develop your resilience to stressful conditions by learning coping strategies that relieve your tension and any anxiety because stress causes damage to your cells.

Here are some popular options that are beneficial to your health and wellbeing You can practise meditation, mindfulness, breathing deeply, reading, taking quizzes, learning a new skills or hobbies as well as taking plenty of appropriate exercise such as dancing, palates, or walking and going out into nature as often as possible in gardens, parks or fields. Do things that you enjoy.

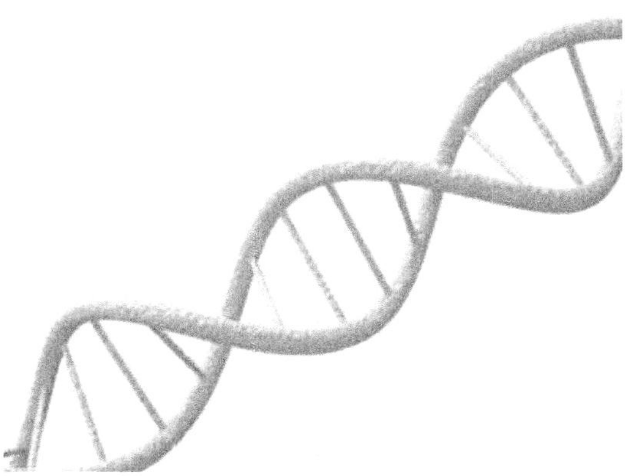

Nutrigenomics

Nutrigenomics involves influencing your genes. Your genes are found within your DNA and have different functions.

The nutrition you put into your body via your diet, is used by the genes as fuel to enable them to carry out their roles. Another way of putting this is that the genes *'express'* themselves.

One way your genes *'express'* themselves is by putting those nutrients back into your body. They put the nutrients into the microsystem in your body. These nutrients are absorbed by your decaying cells and then your cells are rejuvenated and stimulated to reproduce more healthy cells.

The science of nutrigenomics is concerned with controlling your nutrition to suit your individual needs so that you consume foods and drinks specifically for the health benefits that suit your particular genes, your *'genotype'*.

The intention is that once you know your *'genotype'* you are given personalised dietary advice that suits your individual body's requirements and this leads you to make informed choices about the foods that contain the best vitamins and minerals in order for your body to maintain your optimum health and wellbeing.

Epigenomics

Epigenomics also involves intentionally influencing your genes. Remember, your genes lay within your DNA and are there for different purposes. The purpose and role of a gene is referred to as its expression.

Epigenomics involves the study of your *'genome'* (DNA) and involves making changes to your *gene expression* in order to adapt your health condition. This means the performance of the gene is affected and the way it carries out its function is altered.

3 billion pairs of Deoxyribonucleic Acid (DNA) molecules make up 2 strands that coil around each other to form a *'double helix'*, your unique *'genome'*.

This *'genome'* contains the complete genetic code. This is a collection of instructions that are in the blueprint, the plan for your development. This genetic plan of how you grow and how you function, is already planned out and is inside you when you are born into this world. However, inside the *'double helix'* of your DNA there are also 'epigenomes' which are collections of compounds. These occur quite naturally and can interrupt or redirect your DNA. This which means the basic plan of your health can be affected and changed.

Normally, this can be caused by environmental and lifestyle conditions, including stress. Examples of how the environment can affect the way your genes work were found in recent studies concerning post-traumatic stress disorder (PTSD).

It has been shown that people with PTSD who also have high levels of added stress in their work, relationships or lifestyle, have quite different gene expression than those with PTSD but no extra stress. Stress affected the way their genes were expressed and increased the physical signs of ageing and their physical health in those people.

External conditions can trigger chemical responses that create changes however, in epigenomics these changes are purposefully devised and initiated. There is a tremendous amount of research into altering DNA and reprogramming genetic health conditions.

In simple terms, your genes are controlled by turning them on or off. This cannot change your DNA but it can alter your *'gene expression'* and the way your DNS works in your body. This is especially important regarding health conditions that have a genetic cause.

Your Genes and Stress

As I have mentioned before over time stress breaks down your cells decreasing their output of energy into your body. Within each of your cells is a tiny mitochondria which is a *'powerhouse'* of energy. Unfortunately, over time these are attacked by free radicals and as you age these little *'powerhouses'* become depleted and less effective. This causes your cells to decay.

Free radicals are natural chemical by-products created during the activities of your cells. Over time, they eventually overcome the cell and cause it to die. Once the mitochondria inside your cells die, the cells die too. Millions of them stop working and your body becomes less resilient to disease and the signs of ageing set in and become more visible.

You have 46 chromosomes in each of your cells and you have telomeres in your cells that organise the chromosomes and form a protective cover over the end of each chromosome to prevent attacks by free radicals. These shields over the ends of the chromosomes save them decay, from the oxidative stress that the free radicals cause.

Free radicals can also attack your telomeres which divide themselves to conserve their numbers. However, each time your telomeres divide they become shorter and eventually they are too short to be any protection against free radicals and oxidisation.

Unfortunately, the effects of being stressed along with an unhelpful diet and lack of physical exercise, also increases the number of free radicals in your body. Over the years, the loss of telomeres to protect your cells also results in greater vulnerability to disease and oxidative stress, degenerative diseases and ageing. Research has shown that women with longer telomeres live longer than those of the same age with shorter ones. This is why it is vital to actively avoid oxidative stress from free radicals and to purposefully increase your antioxidant levels.

If you would like youthful vitality and health with the lifestyle you want in your latter years you can increase your levels of anti-oxidants through diet, exercise and by building resilience to stressful conditions. Participation in our own health is primarily your own responsibility.

Sirtuins

Sirtuins are causing a great deal of interest because they are critically important in the ageing process. Sirtuins respond to oxidative stress and genotoxic stress by cleaning up your DNA and can turn your genes on and off in this process. Sirtuins are necessary to DNA repair by controlling and antioxidation and inflammation.

However, by the age of 50 your sirtuins lose energy and they become less effective which means you have greater likelihood of inflammation and inflammatory diseases. Most common cause of death in women in the UK is heart disease and vascular dementia which are inflammatory diseases.

There is a huge amount of research focused on sirtuins right now and it has already been found that the decrease in the effectiveness of sirtuins can be reversed. This can be achieved with lifestyle choices, diet and exercise but what is also exciting is that sirtuins can be safely supplemented and still produce the same results.

Curcumin seems to be particularly helpful in extending the life of your sirtuins and their continued effectiveness promises to lengthen your own lifespan, health and quality of life as you age.

Incredible as it may sound, it is also seriously suggested that intervening to increase our sirtuin levels. may eventually lead to age reversal. One of the areas being researched extensively is that of calorie control and limitation and there is extensive research going on into intermittent fasting and prolonged lifespan.

It is not enough to lower calory intake as nutrition has to be carefully balanced at the same time according to your particular genome and gene expression. You might like to keep yourself aware of developments in the research as it is currently suggested that life enhancing solutions will be available within a few years.

Telomeres

Telomeres *(tel-o-meers)* are long segmented strands of DNA that form a protective coating at the end of each one of your chromosomes. Over time the segments disintegrate and cannot be repaired or replaced therefore, your telomeres slowly become shorter and less effective at protecting the end of your chromosomes.

The importance of your telomeres is that their length shows your biological age which is different from your chronological age. Long term studies of telomeres and one study in the UK involving half a million people, have shown that people who walk quickly throughout their life have longer telomeres than people who walk slowly or do not walk much at all. This means that a lifetime of brisk walking can slow down the deterioration of your telomeres and that you can have as much as 16 years longer lifespan simply by taking regular, brisk walks and walking in general, has a positive effect on your longevity.

****

Our future health and experience of ageing is becoming more positive as the science improves and will be very different for our children and their children. The emphasis will be on self-care and taking responsibility for our optimising our own health and the growing understanding of genetics will transform medical interventions.

Ultimately, having a longer lifespan does not have to be a negative experience as it can also give you the potential for a much brighter life in your mature years than you imagined when you were younger.

~ Healthier Living ~

Menopause And Ageing

What is Menopause?

The World Health Organisation (WHO) in 2020, stated that '*natural menopause occurs when a woman has stopped having periods completely, with a clear no show for 12 months.*'

According to the National Health Service (NHS) 2021, British women experience natural menopause between 45 and 55 years of age and the average age is 51 years with 1 in 100 women experiencing premature menopause before the age of 40 and is generally, caused by medical reasons.

Perimenopause is the time either side of menopause when a woman's body is preparing for her fertility to stop or coping with the hormonal changes after she has finished her menstruation completely. This confusing transition stage can last for several years before and after menopause.

At the time of writing this book, only 55,000 are on HRT yet 16,000,000 women in the UK are menopausal and although women experience menopause differently there are many recommendations that more women should be able to have HRT if they choose it.

You cannot predict how long or how severe this may be but the symptoms of being menopausal and preparing for a non-childbearing years, usually persist for about 4 years after your last period but for 1 in 10 women it can continue for as long as 12 years.

Common Symptoms

Hidden, Only You Know

Irregular and stopped periods
Heavy blood loss
Headache
Blurred vision
Tinnitus/Vertigo
Muscle/joint pain
Itchy skin
Vaginal dryness/itching
Painful/uncomfortable sex

Obvious, Others Know

Night sweats
Hot flushes
Mood fluctuations
Fatigue
Weight gain
Thinning hair
Lack of motivation
Weak concentration

Medical, Your Doctor Knows

Urinary tract infections
Thrush/cystitis
Anxiety/depression

Seek advice from you doctor or chemist about any of these symptoms and request blood tests.

The Change

Even if a woman says that *"Age is just a number and it does not define me"* she will almost certainly, have a very different attitude to her, natural and unavoidable, menopause. This means that very often she is sending mixed and confused messages to herself as well as to others about how she feels about menopause and ageing.

Perhaps this is not surprising, because for every day after puberty, she is reminded that she is somewhere within a regular monthly *'cycle'* and so the fluctuating condition of her body; how it feels young and vital one week and how it feels old and sluggish the next is a monthly challenge that goes on for many years.

Even though she would love to be free from the discomfort and inconvenience of menstruation every 28-30 days, mentioning menopause and the end of her menstruation to a woman will usually conjure up mixed feelings for her. Loss of fertility is a big issue for many women but it also involves her assumption and concerns about her attractiveness fading. A woman's confidence and self-esteem can quickly decrease as her images of growing old are far from positive. When fear of losing her femininity and youthfulness is aroused she is likely to attempt to delay the expected physical decline by taking hormone replacement therapy (HRT).

A woman's biological life is complicated but just for now, let us look at the standard, expected experience for most women once their monthly menstruations begin. When you look back in time, history shows us that the number of years that women originally menstruated throughout their lives was very low. Almost all girls married in their very early teens and were almost constantly pregnant which meant they had few periods. Also, as most women back in history did not live long beyond the age of 35-40 menopause was not automatically the common experience it is these days.

Eventually, with improved health care and lifestyle changes women now live longer. This means their fertile years were extended and consequently women now experience more periods and menopause. 21st Century women in many societies benefit from modern science and use birth control to have smaller families. They are also far more likely to have later pregnancies now and can choose to delay pregnancy until much later and be older when they have their first baby. This means they now have far fewer pregnancies compared to all previous generations but they tend to experience more periods and menopause lasts longer more than previous generations throughout history.

Women in the first half of the 20th Century, the world war generations, had little control over their fertility and family size and although they saw menopause as a sign of old age and therefore, an eventual relief from pregnancy they also saw it as a perilous time when, because of their irregular periods, they could so easily find themselves having babies at the same time as their eldest daughters. Many women back then, became pregnant during those unsafe years of perimenopause and menopause.

This also meant that some women were raising young children during and after their menopause and also experiencing later birth. This meant that after years of childbirth women commonly had babies that were often weaker and at greater risk of being born with disabilities. It was also common in those days, for grandmothers to raise grandchildren alongside their own child and for grandchildren to have uncles and aunts of similar ages to themselves. However, being older mothers, enduring labour meant more risk of complications and high death rates for these women. Menopause gave many women cause for concern about unwanted pregnancy especially as contraception if available, was not very successful.

Currently, the majority of ladies in their 60'and 70's in the UK have experienced unprecedented societal and legislative changes. Born after WW2 between 1946 and 1964, these *'baby boomers'* have benefited from healthcare, birth control, higher incomes, greater employment options and better lifestyles. Therefore, these women, their daughters and granddaughters have been able to make quite different decisions about their life paths and their bodies than any of their previous counterparts. The ways they approach their fertility and their menopause is from positions of choice and empowerment that were previously impossible.

The main difference in modern women's menstrual health is they can now choose to delay or avoid menopausal symptoms with interventions such as hormone replacement therapy (HRT). These days, women tend to have mixed feelings about their menstruation. The majority of ladies I coach tell me that although they are a nuisance, their periods are also a positive and welcome sign of fertility and youth. These same ladies often hold negative views about menopause and tend to want to avoid it as they think of it as a sign of ageing which leads to the loss of their sexual attractiveness and vitality.

Modern women have experienced an unprecedented era of control over their fertility, their health and their wellbeing and this has led them to want and expect more from life than any other previous generations.

What is Perimenopause?

To be perimenopausal means you are around the time of menopause and this can be before, during or after your periods stop. Perimenopause is usually associated with the years before menopause but it can also include the years following your last ever period. Changes in your cycle and hormones deficiency can appear in perfectly healthy women before or after menopause but can lead to a wide variety of unwanted symptoms that can be confusing.

1 in 100 women in the UK experience early menopause in their early 40's. This can be for a variety of reasons and it is now suggested that women should learn about and begin to monitor their periods from this age. This can help them avoid mis-diagnosis if they have evidence of changes in their cycle and other symptoms that should highlight menopause to medical professionals. At this earlier age there can be drops in hormones levels and therefore, HRT can be offered to maintain or restore the balance during what can be many years before or after actual menopause.

Common Treatments

In attempts to relieve symptoms, popular medical therapies for menopausal symptoms are hormone replacement therapy, (HRT) counselling and cognitive behavioural therapy (CBT). Alternative and complimentary therapies are also beneficial such as yoga, meditation and enhanced diet and sleep, appropriate exercise and stress management and resilience.

There are a range of effects involved in using different forms of HRT some are beneficial whilst others are harmful therefore, it is an important discussion to have with your doctor.

One aspect often overlooked when embarking on HRT is that within 1 or 2 years and possibly several years longer in some cases, you may want to stop taking it. Although, some women have no further issues many others are shocked when they unexpectedly find they experience the same menopausal symptoms they tried to avoid. However, they can have successfully delayed the effects of menopause and also gained some health benefits from the intervention. This again is an important aspect to discuss with your doctor as medical advice differs greatly and the risks vary so your own individual medical history needs to be considered as well as your personal reasons for wishing to take HRT.

According to prominent consultants Dr Louise Newson and Dr Rebecca Lewis, *'The safest types of HRT are body identical hormones, which means that they are the same structure as the hormones you naturally produce in your body'*. These are regulated whereas HRT based on bio-identical hormones are not regulated.

Therefore, you need to ask questions and look into which types of HRT you are being offered if you choose this method of support.

Other beneficial strategies that have gained popularity that you can practise without side effects are meditation, mindfulness, breathing deeply, stretching your mind by reading, taking quizzes, keeping journals, learning a new skills or hobbies, as well as taking plenty of appropriate exercise such as sport, dancing, pilates, yoga, or walking.

It is important for you to do things that make you happy and that you enjoy. Go out into nature as often as possible in gardens, parks or fields because managing your stress relieves symptoms and also prevents unnecessary ageing. Having the facts about how menopause causes premature ageing is empowering because you can take action to preserve your skin from dehydration and hormonal changes and manage the signs and symptoms such as memory loss and loss of libido and energy.

"I see menopause as the start of the next fabulous phase of life as a woman. Now is a time to 'tune in' to our bodies and embrace this new chapter."

"If anything, I feel more myself and love my body more now, at 58 years old, than ever before."

Kim Cattrall
Actress

Healthy Longevity

Your Physical Health

Nourishment and Movement

During one of my workshops when I asked for a sentence that summed up the experience of growing older, one woman clearly stated, *"For me, it is not a question of which part of my body hurts, it is which part does NOT hurt?"* and almost every woman in the room made noises of agreement.

So, what was going on? What was she experiencing and why was there such a lot of empathy and support for her statement? If it is a common experience for older ladies, why is this?

Most of us expect our bodies to be weaker and to ache as we grow older, but if there is nothing serious diagnosed, then few of us expect to feel so much discomfort.

You have read about epigenetics and nutrigenetics and the inflammation of joints that are caused over time by free radicals and oxidative stress. I recommend you research remedies that can kick starting your Nrf2 pathways and increase your production of antioxidants; however, there are also other ways to improve your overall wellbeing.

Even if you know lots of these, I know many of you have too many distractions and demands on your time, to regularly follow through with your goals to improve your health. Therefore, before you criticise yourself about this, relax. You have probably spent your life putting the needs of others before your own and it is still extremely easy to neglect your own personal self-care simply because it has become a habit to do so.

What can you do to preserve your good health and youthful vitality?

To begin, assess your current physical health.

Nourishment

Starting with the fuel your body needs to maintain health, consider how much water or liquid you drink in a day. Your water intake depends upon the climate you live in. For example, in the UK which has a temperate climate the suggested amount of water per day for an adult is at least 6 glasses 1.2 litres a day and the water in food and beverages is included in this amount. Consider how much water or liquid you consume in a day.

People in affluent countries mostly eat for pleasure so, think about it. What is your main driving factor when it comes to making your food choices?

Do you eat because you enjoy flavours and textures?

Do you eat because you believe you should?

Do you eat because you do not like the feeling of hunger?

Do you eat because you are bored or feeling emotional?

Do you eat to give nutrients to your body?

Nutrition or pleasure?

Consider how much food and what types of food groups you consume in a day, a week and a month. Looking at your answers to the questions and consider what your primary motivation is when you choose your meals. Is it to supply your body with nutrients or is to fulfil your senses and to give you pleasure? Do you eat to avoid hunger or to avoid emotional discomfort? Do you mask your pain with temporary feelings of satisfaction and pleasure?

During food scarcity such as in wars and droughts, people's primary reason for eating is for survival and nourishment and whenever food is difficult to find or it is rationed then meals are planned and scheduled. However, when there is plenty of choice many people's most important motivation for choosing their food is often for self-indulgence instead of its nutritional value.

Modern society is victim to all kinds of deficiencies and gut health problems. Your gut health is also a big influence on your wellbeing, mental health, happiness and longevity. Simply by adding more vegetables and legumes and feeding your gut bacteria well can increase your good health and can add years to life.

I suggest that if you want to feel better and look younger that you improve one area of your diet at a time. For example, if you want to cut down on sugar intake try substituting a biscuit for a banana once a day. This works with children and will work with you too. So, be easy with yourself and be open to new foods and recipes.

Movement

Moving more is proven to increase your vitality and energy especially walking and doing any weight bearing activity. However, there are other benefits including giving your emotions a boost and helping you to be positive and happier. The mental health benefits are now well known, particularly when you walk in amongst nature such as in woodland and forest or by the sea and water or at least in a local park or in gardens.

You saw previously, that having a lifestyle that includes brisk walking helps your telomeres stay long and keep your physical age significantly younger for much longer. Another benefit of regular walking is it helps you to have good quality, longer and deeper sleep which both replenishes and balances your physical, mental and emotional wellbeing.

Next, think about the importance of movement and how much your body needs to maintain agility, stamina and strength. The amount of movement you should do is according to your individual preference and ability.

Do you move more because you enjoy being active?

Do you move because you want a strong, agile and healthy body?

Do you make a point of moving with effort at least every 2 days?

Do you perform your activities with moderate effort?

Do you feel good after you have moved with moderate effort?

Do you deliberately move with intensity at least every 2 days?

Do you feel exhilarated after you have moved with intense effort?

There are 3 main types of movement that are generally advised.

1. Simply take a gentle walk twice a week or perform daily activities such as light housework or pottering in your garden. This is the minimum amount of movement that can be effective and can help you increase your overall health.

2. Do activities that specifically improve your balance, flexibility and strength such as pilates, yoga, stretching, lifting weights or using a resistance band.

If possible, you can build this up to about 2.5 hours over a week of more movement and then you can add more effort such as cycling, dancing, walking, swimming and other sports if you want to.

3. Increase your effort slowly to include more vigorous movement but shorten the amount of time to 75 minutes This could be running, speed swimming, aerobic workout and other fast-moving sports such as squash if it suits you.

High Intensity Interval Training (HIIT) is another strategy. This involves short bursts of anaerobic exercise followed by short periods of recovery which are slower and less intense to improve your cardiovascular health.

I was very impressed by actress Dame Sheila Hancock when she was talking about preparing for a film involving her climbing a mountain. *"I was about 83 and I realised I was' old'. Up until then it hadn't entered my head that I was 'old'. The marvellous thing is that you can get fit no matter how old you are. If you work at it."*

You do not have to climb a mountain but any of these levels of movement will help you to be stronger, improve your balance and increase your agility. Other effects of these activities are that your overall general health is better and your mental and emotional health is also improved.

If you are already active and fit then continuc to maintain these levels of activity as it will help sustain your body. Movement is an important part of your health and your success.

Movement Affirmation

Repeat this affirmation to move easier and build strength with flexibility.

I can move as much as I can

until

I can move as much as I want

Sleep Yourself Young

Sleep

Assess how well your body maintains your good health by taking a moment to consider how much deep sleep you enjoy in a 24-hour period, a week and a month.

It is generally accepted that adults need between 7-9 hours of good quality uninterrupted deep sleep every night.

Do you sleep because you like waking up refreshed?

Do you sleep at set times?

Do you sleep because you do not like feeling tired?

Do you sleep because you are bored or feel emotional?

Do you sleep because your body needs it?

Do you worry about sleeping enough?

Consider how much sleep and the quality of sleep, you have each night, each week and each month. Looking at your answers to the questions, what is your most common experience of sleeping? How often do you sleep? More importantly, how often do you feel completely rested?

What is Sleep?

During sleep your cells repair themselves and your brain produces dreams to make sense of your experiences. To experience complete rest your brain goes through various levels of awareness as you go down into a deep sleep.

Beta level is when you are fully alert and awake.

Alpha level is when you are relaxed and calm, not thinking.

Theta level is when you are deeply relaxed and can visualise and imagine or experience images in the form of dreams with rapid eye movement. (REM).

Delta level is when you are in your deepest, unconscious state and find it difficult to wake up.

Ideally, once you have finished your sleep you should travel back up through these 4 levels of consciousness to full wakefulness and feel fully revitalised and ready to wake up easily.

You have a natural inner clock that informs your brain of when you should sleep and when you should wake up. Each 24 hours is 1 circadian cycle which responds to sunlight. For example, when you are sitting still even if you are watching TV your brain still notices the subtle changes of light at twilight and prepares you to sleep by triggering the release of stress relieving hormones such as dopamine and the *'happy hormone'* serotonin. This creates a cocktail of peaceful chemicals to help you fall asleep.

However, between 1-2am hormones that stimulate your thyroid are released and these can arouse you to wake up at this time. Your metabolism can be disrupted by this and create poor sleep patterns which can be detrimental to your health and lead to weight gain.

Also, research has also shown that a shallow sleep prevents you from reaching Theta level where you normally experience rapid eye movement (REM) and dreams. Studies have shown that this is highly detrimental to your mental and emotional wellbeing.

REM and dream state begins after about 90 minutes of sleep and whilst dreaming does not need to be remembered it does need to be experienced at least 3-5 times during a period of sleep.

The first REM takes about 10 minutes to complete and the last one can last about an hour. Research shows that 25% of all sleep should ideally be spent in REM dream state. This is why 7-9 hours without interruption is so important for a healthy night's sleep.

Sleep Deprivation

Without deep sleep, your energy levels drop and you can easily feel stressed and short tempered. Your health is undermined by poor quality sleep and disrupted patterns because without rest your organs are overworked and your mind becomes less creative. Without enough sleep you are more likely to be pessimistic, less cooperative and angry. Your manner is slower and your energy levels fluctuate and you become forgetful, easily confused and unreliable.

This also affects your facial expressions and you can look aggressive and unapproachable because your face is tense and you smile less and frown more. You can also look tired as your face muscles can drop and your eyes can become dull. Your posture, including walking, standing and sitting and your general vitality can become sluggish and your response times when driving and handling machinery is slower. This is all visible to others around you and can impact them and their opinion of you.

Never underestimate your need for good quality sleep.

Sleep Yourself Well

Your Circadian Clock

Your body's *'internal clock'* system runs on a 24-hour cycle and your body is influenced by the sun and daylight hours. The primary stress hormone cortisol, signals to your brain that it is daytime and makes you alert. It wakes you up or it prevents you from falling asleep altogether. Any sleep schedule that does not give you enough deep sleep confuses your body and if you cannot sleep when you need to it can lead to health problems.

If you wake up regularly throughout the night and have poorer quality and less sleep than you used to then you are likely to feel tired and lack energy throughout your day. This means you may need a 'power nap' to help you keep going. Researchers have also found that sleep deprivation alters the levels of endocannabinoid in your brain which activate your brain's *'reward system' because* Endocannabinoid stimulates your thyroid and your metabolic rate and this hormone also affects your appetite. Poor sleep affects your metabolism and motivates you to indulge in midnight snacks or early morning biscuits which results you gaining unwanted weight.

Your Thyroid

Leptin and ghrelin are hormones regulate your feelings of hunger and your feelings of being full. Leptin supresses hunger whereas ghrelin is the *'hunger hormone'*. Every night between 1-2am ghrelin stimulates your thyroid and this makes you ready to wake up and look for a snack.

When you do not sleep at night you lose energy and your body uses up its store of energy from the meals you ate during the day. To make sure you have enough energy your thyroid and your adrenal glands work together. However, if your thyroid does not work properly, your adrenal glands produce more adrenalin and cortisol which is known as the *'stress hormone'* but the adrenalin keeps you awake.

Therefore, you are more likely to eat during the night and more likely to put on extra weight. If you have sleep problems and fatigue you should check your problems with your doctor.

Cleaning Your Brain

You need to enjoy a good sleep and to sleep well for as long as you can without disruption because it gives your brain time to *'clean'* itself up every night.

Your body has a glymphatic system which helps to remove a toxic protein, beta-amyloid from your brain. Beta-amyloid is a toxin gathers in your brain but what is disturbing is that it is found in abundance in the brains of people with Alzheimer's disease.

When you sleep, beta-amyloid is quickly cleared away but when you are awake it is cleared very slowly. Therefore, when your sleep is disrupted this sleep deprivation prevents your brain from performing its daily *'clean up'* and removal of these toxic proteins. Lack of sleep leaves your brain full of toxins whereas sleep keeps your brain healthy.

Sleep Well to be Well

Regular, deep sleep for 7-9 hours has been shown to –

Reduce the risk of
* type 2 diabetes.
* cardiovascular disease.
* certain types of cancer.

Maintains healthy weight by
* managing hunger hormones.
* turning off reward centre in your brain.
* reducing calorie intake especially via sugary snacks.

Physical Health

Good physical health is linked to fitness and performing the physical tasks involved in life well. Being fit and healthy helps you look and feel young and certainly helps with fewer illnesses, diseases and injuries.

- Choose a physical activity you enjoy and do it often.
- Develop good balance, co-ordination and agility.
- Build up your strength, flexibility and stamina.

Mental and Emotional Health

Good mental and emotional health is closely linked to your personal wellbeing and feeling positive about your future. Having faith and belief in yourself keeps you cheerful and focused on solutions. You also become clear minded and think constructive thoughts. Life is easier with a happy outlook.

This also includes developing your emotional intelligence and in my view, your emotional health involves living a life of wellbeing, balance and contentment, which means you become resourceful and resilient.

According to the World Health Organisation, (WHO), health is **'...** *a state of complete physical, mental and social well- being...'*

WHO also states that you have mental health when you *'...can cope with the normal stresses of life, can work productively and fruitfully'* and you *'...can contribute to your community?'*

As stated by the BBC, 'Being emotionally healthy includes Social health which also contributes to wellbeing. It is feeling positive about yourself and feeling positive about interactions with other people and the wider world.'

Emotional health is not usually considered separately but professionals would generally agree with these ideas of what emotional health is. *'Emotional health is when you can identify and understand the range of feelings you have and appreciate their value.'*

However, this does not mean that you should accept negative emotions if they overwhelm you. Emotional health also involves your attitude to your emotions and your reactions including your attitude to your behaviours and whether you can restrain yourself.

Every 7 days, choose one of these to practise for a whole week.

- Accept and respect yourself, your qualities and your skills.
- Give yourself permission to be proud of yourself.
- Decide to be optimistic about the future.

- Practise replacing your negative thoughts with positive ones.
- Recognise your feelings but be cautious when and how you express them.
- Give yourself permission to be happy and enjoy it.

Social Health

Associating with other people who welcome and support you is uplifting. Friendly and stimulating experiences that contribute to your wellbeing and develop your confidence are inspiring. Enjoy positive interactions with other people in the wider world as they increase your sense of belonging and makes you feel safe and secure.

Top Tips

to improve your emotional and mental health.

Be Aware
Identify your personal strengths and build them up.

Be Positive
Learn to be optimistic and expect good outcomes from bad situations.

Be Brave
Develop courage and live your life according to your own values.

Be Resilient
Decide to bounce back from setbacks. Learn from them and expect difficulties to open up new possibilities.

Be Self-Caring
Develop a positive self-image and compassionate understanding of yourself.

Be Friendly
Create a social network that supports and encourages you.

Be Clever
Develop a specific set of skills to cope with stress and mental health difficulties and external stress.

Be Focused
Discover a sense of purpose for your life and develop motivation for your activities, projects and adventures.

Be Adventurous
Make time for hobbies, interests and leisure that add quality and value to your life.

Be Proud
All of your achievements and all of your setbacks enrich your life. Every attempt to progress gives you an interesting life so be proud of your effort and your courage.

Healthy Sleep

Sleep gives you relief from stress. It keeps your vitality high and cleans your brain of toxins. When you sleep you fast which gives your liver and kidneys a long rest and this replenishes your cells and rebalances your body.

Looking after your liver and kidneys improves your skin and the brightness of your eyes. Sleep improves your mood and maintains brain function and also helps your mind to sort through your emotions and mental concerns so that you can resolve issues in your dreams.

Stay Healthy, Stay Happy

Keep these factors in mind as you plan your time and find the best ways for you to achieve your goals. For example, if you cannot attend a fitness group or cannot do aerobic exercises then find videos on the internet and if you cannot get out and about then find a social and hobby group on-line.

If you do not have access to internet and technology call your local library, school PTA or religious communities to find groups that can help you. There are always people ready to help and come up with solutions that suit your particular needs so even if it takes a little time speak to people and ask for their ideas.

Top Tips For Great Sleep

1. Prepare your bedroom for sleep only and keep your sleep environment as dark as possible.

2. Review any medications you are taking in case they may interfere with sleep or cause you to sleep during the daytime leaving you alert at night.

3. Use the bathroom often in the hours before bedtime to make yourself comfortable for the night.

4. Before sleeping eat a small banana as it contains muscle relaxing potassium and magnesium or drink a small banana infusion.

5. Try cherries before sleep time as they contain high levels of sleep-inducing melatonin or drink a little cherry infusion.

6. Ease any aches and pains by stretching for a few minutes before getting into bed.

7. Tuck your bedcovers in tight and use heavy blankets to make you feel cosy.

8. If pain or discomfort such as restless leg syndrome (RLS) keeps you awake at night consult your doctor.

You need sleep to maintain your health and success. Here are some extra tips.

1. Make your bedroom a calm and peaceful space.

2. During the day get out into as much natural sunlight as possible.

3. Move more energetically during the day and get up after every hour of sitting.

4. Limit caffeine, nicotine, alcohol and big meals in the evening.

5. Stop using any bright screens 2 hours before going to bed.

6. Choose only relaxing activities before sleep.

7. Set timer so that you go to bed and get up at the same times every day.

Sleep deeper and enjoy a great healing rest with this affirmation

Say it **complete or split** it in half for the morning and evening.

Say it out loud or say it quietly to yourself often every day.

Say it in the morning and at lunch time when you stop to rest and take nourishment.

Say it at night-time before you sleep.

Say it often, many times more and make it a habit.

I sleep deeply anywhere, anytime I like for as long as I want

I can sleep when I want, where I want as often as I want

Ladies In Weighting

Why Does Weight Increase as Age Increases?

Surveys show that many women aged over 50 years old believe that being overweight is one reason they may become seriously ill and could be the reason they may die early because they often see it as a precursor to diabetes and heart disease. They often dread being looked upon as a burden and a drain on family, friends and medical resources and they also worry that being overweight at any age carries a stigma which is heightened as we grow older and this leads to them have low self-esteem and lack of confidence.

Here are some of the theories that research shows may cause your weight to go up, as your age goes up. Sometimes, there is very little we can do about it but awareness is half the cure. Stigma and prejudice about being overweight can disappear if any of the following research results resonate with you.

Identify Your Set Point?

Research has shown that under normal circumstances you have an inbuilt biological process that regulates your weight, a *Set Point.* This means there is a specific weight that your body prefers. This *Set Point* occurs according to your individual make-up and which of the different stages and ages of your life you are in at the time. These stages are Pre-Puberty, Post-Puberty, Fertility, Peri-Menopause, Menopause and Post-Menopause.

Example 1. Pre-puberty, you may be a thin child but post-puberty you can find your shape and weight are more different than you might expect. This is okay though because you can even put on 5lbs over the winter and lose it without effort in the spring. No one says anything about your weight.

Example 2. You maintain the same weight all your life until you have babies. For a few years your weight fluctuates and after a while you have gained a lot of weight. You can lose it sometimes but then put it on again. You maintain that weight gain of a couple of stone than before no matter what you do. Others give you a lot of sympathy and encouragement.

Example 3. Throughout life, you may gain weight or you may lose weight. This is okay though because you can drop the pounds with diet and exercise. After *menopause,* you put weight on and on until it moves up a stone or two but this is still okay because you accept your 'normal' weight has just moved up. You accept this is the new version of you but you move between the following three attitudes.

a) You may resist the weight gain and push yourself go to the gym, watch your diet and worry about your clothes fitting.

b) You may beat yourself up about looking like your mother and feeling old so you are grumpy and often cry when you look in your wardrobe. You miss your old self and how you used to look.

c) You may accept your weight but stay as healthy as possible and you get on with your life.

In simple terms, each stage that your body goes through has an optimum weight and body shape that is best for your health and performance and it is set to suit your individual physical blueprint. This is why so many ladies put weight on in specific areas such as their waist and tummy after menopause. Research shows your *Set Point* exists to protect your health and give you longevity.

Your Settling Point

Your weight responds to how, when and where you nourish it and use it. Therefore, your weight can fluctuate to any level at any age and stay at that level until something changes to affect it. This type of weight gain depends on factors such as environment and availability of certain foods and opportunity to take exercise or not.

Your weight changes throughout your life and appears to have no regular pattern as it is gained and lost because of a range of influences. For example, if you take a job where you often attended dinner functions you gain weight and keep it on until 5years later you learn a new sport and are more active. You lose weight and this then stays your constant weight for several years. Later, you have a knee injury and stop all sport but you join a cake-making class and enjoy eating your creations. This time you gain weight and maintain that weight for a number of years.

Your activity, your behaviour, your environment and your culture all impact your weight and your body *'settles'* into your weight at that time until something changes either way.

Your Dual Intervention Point

Your body has both a *Set Point* and a *Settling Point.* The Intervention Point is when your body overrides the *Set Point* and goes towards the *Settling Point.* You can rely on your body to regulate your weight for your optimum health.

However, modern life undermines your health in many ways and your weight is often one of the ways life puts your health in jeopardy.

Here is a common example.

Your *Set Point* fluctuates but your *Intervention Point* stops the fluctuation enabling your body to reach a *Settling Point* where the weight stays the same for a period of time and eventually this is then your new *Set Point.*

For example, you have been active and busy all your life but you have turned 55years old and decided to take a less physically demanding job with less commuting. You change your job to a more sedentary role working at a desk but colleagues often bring cakes in to share and generally there is a lot more socialising at lunch times than you are used to.

Imagine that up until this job change your body has a weight *Set Point* at 10stone but the change of habits in your new job create extra weight gain. This increase in weight fluctuates depending on celebrations, season and emotional upsets and stress.

The weight gain continues until your body weighs 12stone and you may become a *'yoyo dieter'* in your efforts to control your weight.

This is when your body decides you have reached the *Intervention Point* and stops the up and down weight situation because it makes your vital organs work harder and is unhealthy.

Your body then relaxes into one weight; a *Settling Point* and finds the most healthy level of weight for you to maintain in those working conditions.

When the weight gain settles then that becomes the new normal weight for you. In this example the new Set Point of 11stone is fixed and becomes your new *Set Point.*

As a woman, there are certain stages of your life such as menopause during which you can put weight on despite your own best efforts. You may feel frustrated and disheartened when your weight fluctuations eventually become fixed at a new *Set Point* that is heavier than you had before.

Are you are concerned about your health, your longevity and your enjoyment of life as you grow older?

When it comes to it, one size does not fit all and no single health model is going to perfectly explain why some maintain their ideal weight and others simply do not.

Despite what you may believe about being overweight it has been proven in more than one study that *slightly* heavier women live longer than their average-weight or under-weight counterparts.

Now this seems counter-intuitive but in studies by Dr K. Flegal, when overweight and *slightly* obese women experience any life threatening medical conditions and diseases they are far more likely to recover.

In further studies, *heavier* women are found to live longer but they live with more illness and endure more serious health problems.

According to Dr J. Mitteldorf, women who lived the longest were of *average weight* when they were young but *overweight* in their later years and once they were post menopause.

Generally, an increase in weight as you age may not be pleasing but it does appear to be nature's way of helping you to survive and although, there can be health risks it is still more likely to mean that you can have a long and happy life.

After a series of operations many years ago, I remember a nurse telling me that being a bit heavier as we mature was an advantage because being underweight in old age often meant the body had no reserves to use up during some illnesses. At the time, I was not impressed by this viewpoint as I had a slim body all my young life and did not ever imagine that I would put weight on.

"The best role models for women are people who are themselves and who bring light to the world."

"What makes you different is your strength."

Emma Thompson
Actress, Author, Producer and Activist

~ Wanting More ~

Your Purpose: A Meaningful Life

Feeling Invisible and Wanting More

Many mature women have a belief that they should be pursuing some specific purpose. They sense that they are meant to be someone more than they are and be doing something special in their life but they often give up on finding their purpose and developing it.

Some ladies already have a burning desire to pursue a purpose but feel frustrated with life and themselves because they have not achieved all that they believe they are or were capable of.

Some women lose motivation as they get older and feel they are drifting aimlessly through life. They wish they could be excited and focused again but they struggle to regard anything they want to do as having any value anymore.

Clients often tell me they believe it is all too late for them and they question who would be interested and who would listen or take notice of them. They also ask whether they are being selfish or not.

Being self-motivated is not a negative thing for any woman. Sacrificing your own needs and becoming depleted of physical energy and mental wellbeing does not help others and does not help you. Even mothers must take care of themselves if their children are going to be safe and thrive. However, women deal with a continual juggling act between their own needs and the needs of others who depend on them.

As a mature woman you can often find that you either have total focus and courageously forge your way ahead or you can lack the confidence to pursue any of your own needs at all. Perhaps, you switch between the two and find this only creates confusion.

With a long life expectancy, you may decide to use your *'Seenager'* years to achieve more of your potential and you might try new things but several situations seem to keep you in your current status quo.

Your choices can cause family, friends and colleagues to make negative comments about your ideas and goals which may cause you to doubt yourself. You may experience loss of self-esteem if or when you give up your employment to retire because although it is a pleasure to be at home you may feel redundant and useless.

You might also feel you have lost sight of yourself as an individual by taking on extra family responsibilities and becoming enmeshed in other people's needs once again. You may have come to the conclusion that you have existed solely as an extension to other people's ideas about what your life should be like and this can make you feel rebellious.

This can be the time you that you realise you want a life of your own but you are likely to find yourself in the *'sandwich years'* looking after both parents and grandchildren and sharing your resources with them to help the out.

It is not all bad though because loving grandchildren and helping children raise their families makes you feel valued and this has great rewards. However, clients often tell me that they feel lost and incapable of making some important changes. They do not believe they have the power to achieve things they have always wanted to do and willingly sacrifice their own dreams for their family.

Not only do they believe they cannot achieve their purpose but quite often they do not know what that even is yet. They need time to find themselves and their vision but life sweeps them along.

It is often easier for women to continue to help others fulfil their dreams and goals and put their own dreams aside. Giving up is an option but my clients question the quality of their lives and their health and are aware that they are likely to have more time and longevity but they need help to maintain their hope for their future dreams.

When you are feeling like this you may find you are unable to hold on to thoughts and ideas as they seem to quickly flow into each other or maybe they disappear as soon as they appear and are quickly replaced by doubts and anxiety. It can seem as if you cannot control this internal dialogue or internal current of emotional churning.

However, rather than being a sign of a frail mind, dementia or declining faculties, it is much more likely to be caused by stress and possibly anxiety.

Therefore, it is important that you believe in yourself and understand that you do not have to spend the next phase of your life frustrated or disappointed, consumed by worry about your future.

Women also tell me that even if they can reorganise their family commitments they do not have the resources, the finance, the time to take risks but this is often due to a lack of clarity. It is this lack of clarity that often limits their vision and they have difficulty believing that all barriers and obstacles are insurmountable. They need help to see their way forward clearly and to make a plan that works for them in their individual situations.

I assure you that as each age brings both challenges and rewards. When you focus on your blessings and embrace all the positives, you can be thrilled by your new opportunities. Stay optimistic and practise being relaxed and patient whilst you put the life you want together and bring it into your reality. It may start off slowly but it picks up momentum and you can change things for the better without feelings of guilt. It is possible and you CAN find the balance and fulfilment you want.

Your Purpose, Your Passion

Perhaps you do not have a strong sense of purpose and maybe you are happy to take life as it comes. This may mean you are content right now to be reactive and not proactive. You do not have to drive your life forward.

We all have times in life when we are not proactive. It is all good. I know many women in this mode and I believe it is a good and healthy way to be in most cases and is often a resting phase as you wait and prepare for something new to occur or you wait for an urge to arise from within you.

This can be a valuable period and only you know when you are ready. Like the caterpillar in the chrysalis, you may simply be waiting for the right time to be rejuvenated and to wake up become a 'Seenager' *and* show the world your transformation.

So, what is *'purpose'*? According to most dictionaries having a purpose is about focusing on an outcome and moving towards a desired result and achieving a specific goal. It is usually having a desired dream such as expressing your talent, skill, creativity or by significantly changing direction. Examples of this could be opening a shop, writing hit songs, putting on an art exhibition, running a marathon, learning to dance, playing an instrument or studying for a university degree.

However, if this seems to be too much of a leap there are many smaller steps to be taken first which involve decisions and actions that can lead you steadily toward your goals. For example, if you want to be successful in business, you need to start and learn how to establish and grow your business. If you want to go traveling then you need to plan your transport, route and equipment. If you want a relationship with a new love then you need to invest in some clothes, social events and possibly a dating site. All these initial steps build your confidence as you work towards your ultimate fulfilment.

Decide what your purpose is and what you think that will look like once you have achieved it. You need to decide this first because knowing what your purpose is, motivates you to move forwards even when things are not working out, until you eventually succeed.

Your purpose can also be defined as a sense of '*life purpose'*, which is a sense of being connected to a greater or higher ideal. Women frequently tell me they feel they have a religious calling or political vocation or maybe they have always wanted to save animals and set up a sanctuary. There are so many ideas because they are wonderful souls with so much to offer the world and you are also full of potential.

This usually means you have a sense of responsibility and again this can cause feeling of guilt in you if you believe you are not fulfilling your purpose. Therefore, you may worry if you do not have a sense of what your purpose is or that you are not achieving what you think you *'should'* be doing, Your worst fear may be that your life and your potential has been, still is being and is going to continue to be wasted.

Ultimately, you need to be ready when the opportunities you want appear in your life. Remember, you have many healthy exciting years ahead with plenty of time to enjoy and achieve more than you ever think you can.

If there is anything specific stopping you, here is my mantra for you to repeat. Sit quietly, breathe deeply and relax then repeat this mantra either out aloud or quietly to yourself often.

My Purpose Is Known To Me

My Purpose Motivates Me

Redefining Your Identity

I am sure you will agree that you need to understand yourself and know *'who'* you are. This is a big issue for many women but many of my clients find it difficult to define themselves when I ask them, *"Who are you when you are not playing all the roles you have accumulated in life?"*

You may respond by immediately thinking, *"Oh, but I already know who I am and I can't change who I am, nor do I want to"*. This is fine but what you are saying is, you know who you have been so far, in terms of what the world has given you and required of you, up until now. However, do you know, who you can become? Are there parts of yourself you have never expressed or shown the world? Is it possible that there could still be parts of you that you are not aware of yet?

You may believe you can be a better version of *'You'*, a more natural version or perhaps you feel there is a different part of *'You'* that *'should'* be coming forward.

Journalist, TV Host and Author, Lorraine Kelly said in her morning show, *"We are allowed to change and we are allowed to have opinions. We should be allowed to have debates and we should listen to each other. We should be able to hear the other side of things otherwise we never learn anything and we don't grow."*

I agree with her that all of us need to be open minded and so that you can create your own rejuvenation you need to explore ideas that can give meaning to your life and help you to find your sense of purpose.

This is where coaching and working through a specific programme that is adjusted to your own unique life can help by quickening the time and simplifying the struggle, involved in your self-discovery.

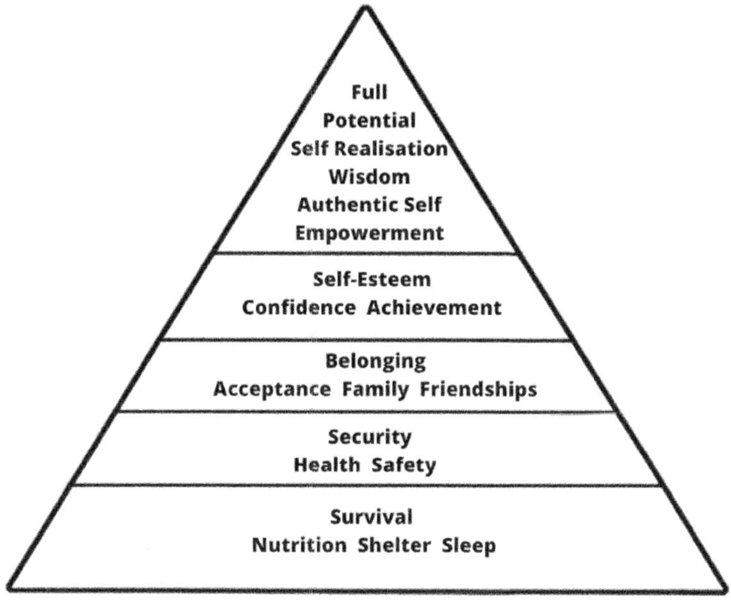

Image by victoriasheridan.com 2022 inspired by Charles D McDermid 1960, based on Abraham Maslow Theory 1943

Identify your own position, at this point in your life.

1. **Are your needs for physical survival**
   Not Met – Partially Met – Mostly Met – Completely Met

2. **Are your needs for personal security**
   Not Met – Partially Met – Mostly Met – Completely Met

3. **Are your needs for being accepted belonging**
   Not Met – Partially Met – Mostly Met – Completely Met

4. **Are your needs for self-esteem and for achieving**
   Not Met – Partially Met – Mostly Met – Completely Met

5. **Are your needs for personal empowerment**
   Not Met – Partially Met – Mostly Met – Completely Met

In his theory Abraham Maslow suggests you move up and down the pyramid but you are more likely to achieve your full potential and eventually transcend their impact on you once all or most levels are satisfied. You may not agree with his ideas but you might find the exercise thought provoking and useful.

Look at your answers on the previous page and think about which needs are not being fully met and what that means for you. Then consider what you require and what needs to happen in order for you to fill those gaps and make it happen.

One of the great things about being a mature woman, a *'Seenager'*, is that you can be freer with more choices than when you were a younger woman. It is possible to rearrange your life and create opportunities so that your passions can flow.

What Does a *'Meaningful Life'* Mean for You?

Yes, you can certainly have a meaningful life without having a sense of purpose but we tend to think the two usually go together. There are many ways to find meaning in the important areas of your life but because having a meaningful purpose is always a very subjective experience I would like you to take time to think and to understand what *'meaningful'* means to you.

Meaning can be the driving force that gives your purpose power. The MEANING you give to your life is based on your VALUES and yet you may not have identified all of your values.

Do this Now

1 **Write a list of your values**, This shows you your *authentic self.* Then you can see if your most meaningful purpose is actually in line with your *authentic self.* After this, you can be confident that your life **purpose has the passion that motivates to achieve** everything you want.

2 **Write a list of all the things you have ever wanted to do**. What do you feel inspired to do? Would love to do? Even if it includes **a big dream**. This is your inner self, your subconscious speaking to your conscious mind.

3 **Allocate your values to each purpose**. This helps you identify which ones are in line with your *authentic self.* These **drive your passion to achieve** They give you a fresh awareness your newfound sense of purpose and help you to be happy.

~ Your Life ~

Your *Values* feed your need for a life full of *Meaning*

The *Meaning* you give to your life gives you, your sense of *Purpose*

Your *Purpose* inspires your *Motivation*

Your *Motivation* leads you to your *Fulfilment*

Values
↓
Meaning → Purpose → Motivation → Fulfilment

‘Seenagers’ In Love

Romance

We are now expected to live until well over 100 years old and therefore significant numbers of us will be spending part of our lives with more than one partner. We can also expect to have our love lives turned upside down as the number of years we spend being older become more than we spend being young.

This means our understanding and expectations of intimate relationships, love and romance are changing.

The modern trends are that more young people are choosing to live alone and more couples are choosing not to have children. If these trends continue this could have a big effect on lifestyle in later life and how future generations experience their longevity.

Meanwhile, for those of us just entering or already in our later years more of us ladies are also choosing to live alone. This does not mean we do not want companionship and romance with someone special to love and care about us. However, it does appear that older women now prefer to have the benefits of a relationship without the disadvantages and are choosing to keep separate homes.

This is causing more older men to worry about their futures and studies show that mature men are now finding it difficult to find women who want to cohabitate. This means men are feeling less loved and cared for than they are used to which is leading to higher cases of loneliness in men than in women who tend to have stronger more supportive friendships and social connections.

Whether women are living with a partner or not, many of us are deciding that age is no barrier to romance and loving relationships and many are discovering that love and companionship in their *'Seenager'* years is just as much fun and just as meaningful as when they were teenagers. We can all be *'Seenagers'* again but with wisdom gained from life's experiences.

Most older women entering new relationships believe they must support others to be happy; however, many are now realising that they now need to look after and fulfil themselves first in order to be happy in a relationship.

1. Consider your own personal beliefs about this because you will find greater happiness if you identify the beliefs that underpin and reinforce your expectations. Then decide whether they serve you well or not before you embark on a new relationship.

2. Think about your values and ask yourself if your life reflects those values. Are they based on your outlook when you were a teenager or a young adult and are they still relevant at this stage of your life?

The Dating Game

Generally, most ladies who come to me ask for help and guidance because they realise they have beliefs that are limiting their progress. Outdated beliefs they have held on to for a long time that are not relevant anymore are often holding them back.

This is frequently true for women who find themselves alone, coming out of divorce or bereavement. After a while they begin to realise they want to spend the rest of their lives with love and companionship and a partner again. However, they may not have dated for decades and very often they do not know how or where to meet a new partner.

When it comes to dating there are usually 2 approaches that are more prevalent One is open and optimistic and often falls in love easily. The other is cautious and cynical with fixed ideas and is frequently unwilling to let go emotionally. In my experience, finding older ladies who have a more balanced and pragmatic approach about dating is not so common but whichever approach they take all women can find wholesome and rewarding relationships at any stage of their lives.

They say things such as, *"How do I act on a date at my age? I'm no teenager. I'm just not attractive anymore, I've lost the looks I had when I was younger. There are younger, more beautiful women. What do I say? What do I do? I don't have a lot of time left. I don't have the confidence. Where do I go to meet someone special?"*

Helping ladies to take the first steps into dating begins with building their confidence and self-esteem. They deserve to have fun and more than that they deserve a loving relationship.

Here are some essential tips for dating someone you met online.

Your First Time Dating ONLINE

7 ways to stay safe.

1. Ask for more photos so you can see they have a real life and are not misleading you about their age and are not using a using a fake profile.

2. Do not share personal information such as family names, jobs, activities until much later if a relationship blooms.

3. Do not give your home address or phone number – use a safe app or email instead.

4. Get to know someone and check what they say is true.
5. When you feel excited it may not be *'love'* so wait to find out more about your feelings.

6. Listen and reflect on flattery and mirroring, e.g., if you say you like a particular band or song and the other person says they like it too, are they being genuine or just flattering you.

7. Never lend or send them money, no matter how little or how urgent.

One of the things I have found, is that many women in this situation often have an idealistic view of what that partner *'should'* be which can lead to difficulty. If you are always asking someone to live up to the image you have of someone else or have a check list of what you want and nothing less will do, then a relationship can be a source of disappointment and further feelings of heart ache.

Sadly, when older women are cynical and over cautious they easily deter any amorous advances. They frequently neglect to fan the flames of new romance and are likely to give up at the first sign of incompatibility. They very often prevent themselves from having the opportunity to step out of their comfort zone and enjoy what life has to offer. I suggest you allow yourself time to at least make a new friend.

It does not matter whether mature women have spent their lives in easy or difficult relationships or what age they are, they can feel like teenagers when they are given attention and romance. They can fall in love with being in love and being romanced. It is surprising how many ladies revert back to their youthful behaviours and unrealistic hopes of a *'knight in shining armour'* coming along to sweep them off their feet and save them from their solitude. It is a beautiful idealistic wish that can make some women very gullible and vulnerable.

'Love is blind' and for some women being a *'Seenager in love'*. can be both amazing and hazardous. The biggest worry that other people, friends and family have for middle-aged women who are looking for love is that they fall in love but are unaware of the of modern pitfalls of dating.

All the wisdom of their years can quickly disappear in the excitement of romantic flattery so caution is needed to make sure it is a real and deep affection that will last.

Take Care of Yourself

Despite years of life experience the same hormones and chemicals come into play in matters of the heart and when they are in love older women have the same hopes, beliefs and expectations as when they were younger women.

The biology of love is the same whether you are younger and older. The *'love'* chemicals such as dopamine, serotonin and oxytocin. These are released by your brain and give you an addictive feeling of bliss and excitement. You are also unlikely to *'run away'* because your stress hormones subside and you are left with feelings desire.

If the person who is the object of your desire is not feeling the same it can leave you open to being taken advantage of and being abused so review your relationship at intervals to check it is authentic and healthy for both of you.

Sexually Transmitted Infections (STI) are rife amongst over 50 year olds so without sounding patronising, I care enough about you to remind you to take care of yourself in every sexual encounter until you are strongly committed to each other.

Being in love can make you idealise the person you desire. You find them exciting and you might trust them in sexual matters before you really know them. Also, if you are in your menopause you may want to take precautions and be careful to also protect yourself against unwanted pregnancy.

Your First Time Dating OUT

5 *Ways To Stay Safe*

1. Meet in a public place not in a car park and do not get in their car to go on somewhere else.

2. Tell a friend or relative the person's details, where you are going, how you are getting there and who you are meeting.

3. Ask your friend to text you during the date and if the person is offended by this then they are not for you.

4. If you do not feel comfortable and you are in a restaurant or bar ask someone who works there to help you or watch you get to your car and leave.

The best advice here is not to become intimate with a stranger until you know them better and you may want to be certain that person is not dating other people before putting your sexual health at risk.

What Happens in the Bedroom?

If you are alone but looking for a new relationship in your later years, you may be confused whether you want company and friendship or a deep loving and committed relationship. You may want your own space to explore your own interests but you might also long for a cuddle or you may want a close intense scenario in which you and your partner are inseparable.

Whatever you want in a relationship, you are likely to think about what the bedroom intimacy will be like and you may have mixed views about it. Ideally, you can still do what comes naturally but many of my clients tell me they worry about the practicalities of intimacy especially if they have any health complications.

Emma Thompson, reflecting on her role as Nancy in the film 'Good Luck To You Leo Grande' said, *"A lot of women look back on their lives and wonder if they've fully experienced what we think of as essential part of life. Shockingly, 15% of women say they have never had an orgasm, even on their own. Women don't own up to not having sexual pleasure and don't know how or where to get it."* They want intimacy but very often they are afraid of it so, being honest and having discussions with partners in a genteel way can help them find the sexual fulfilment they want. Acknowledging your own sexuality is empowering and you want to enjoy your inner desires and closeness within a relationship with care and respect for your body.

If you have any health concerns around sex in a relationship you can speak to a doctor or a practice nurse. Sadly, caution is needed if you are a middle aged woman entering new relationships. Contracting an STI is a serious risk and it is also important to secure your financial position. Falling in love with the wrong person is still a hazard and a strong relationship takes time to ripen. When you are young you are able to rebuild your financial security but it is unlikely that you will be able to do so in your *'Seenager'* years. I suggest you need to be sure of the other person's intentions and hopefully you can resist the urge to rush into a commitment.

You may think its rude to ask your potential bed partner for medical checks such as STD and HIV tests and you may not feel comfortable discussing protection. You are not alone and most mature women do not discuss these matters even though they have concerns. You might not wish to disclose your own information or alternatively, you may well be confident about tackling the subject. Many mature ladies do not have the confidence or experience to be forthright and you may feel uncomfortable about bringing the romance down to basic negotiations. However, for your own health and safety and for your partner's wellbeing too you need to find a way to have this discussion and you can usually find support from friends or clinics to help you with this.

When they begin a new relationship, women are looking for love, romance and friendship but they also want to enjoy the freedom of sex without the fear of unwanted pregnancy. This sense of liberation seems perfect for them to enjoy themselves. It may surprise you to know that women reach a sexual peak just before menopause and their sexual desire is heightened because they are motivated biologically to find a mate before their fertile years are over. This can make older ladies quite passionate and attractive especially to new partners.

During perimenopause and menopause, you may worry that you will lose your libido altogether and that their current or potential partner may be discouraged by this or you may have already reached this stage already. However, this does not happen to every woman but if it does, a couple can learn to arouse each other with love and patience and with a sense of fun and tenderness they can continue to enjoy sex and intimacy in different ways for many years.

Sex can also become a *'no-go area'* as the hormones settle and their bodies go into their non-reproductive state. Whereas there are women who are not content to have romance without sex or some kind of intimacy there are other women who find it easy to stop and say *"No"* to everything.

It may surprise you to know that I have also helped lots of men with stress and anxiety, during which time some of the older men have had told me their anxiety includes issues around sex too. Those men have consistently said that they were often secretly pleased when their women lost interest in sex as it took the pressure off them to perform. They did not want to admit this to their partners let alone their friends and for those men sex was a large source of their anxiety and stress.

As the majority of couples assume that post-menopausal women lose interest in intimacy or have difficulty and discomfort during sex it is easy for men to allow women to accept sole responsibility for lack of activity in the bedroom even though, they have confessed to me that they also have anxiety about having a much lower libido and are relieved when women avoid sex. This conveniently leaves men with their self-esteem and *'macho'* reputation intact.

It is important to know before you start dating or worrying about having sex that many men have their bedroom concerns too and are embarrassed to admit it. Therefore, honest discussion early in your relationship can build trust and confidence to move into the bedroom when you are both ready.

'Love is blind' and for some women being a *'Seenager in love'* can be both amazing and hazardous. Older women have the same hopes, beliefs and expectations as younger women and despite their years of life experience, they have the same hormones and chemicals released that make them feel highly elated.

The biggest worry that other people, friends and family have for middle-aged women who are looking for love is that they fall in love with people they meet on dating sites but are unaware of the of modern pitfalls and the games some people play.

The biology of love is the same whether you are younger and older because the release of *'love'* chemicals such as dopamine and serotonin together with oxytocin give you an addictive feeling of bliss and excitement which can make you a bit obsessive. Also, you tend to be unwilling to run away and eventually, your stress hormones and cortisol subside. This state leaves you with desire and trust in the other person. If the person of your desire is not feeling the same it can leave you open to being taken advantage of and being abused so try to review your relationship at intervals to check it is authentic and healthy for both of you.

Being in love can make you idealise the person you desire. You find them exciting and you might trust them before you really know them. Therefore, if you are in the middle of your menopause you may want to take precautions and be careful to protect yourself of unwanted pregnancy.

8 Ways To Have Fun Dating

1. Make the best of yourself but importantly feel good in what you are wearing.

2. Be confident and value yourself and what you can contribute to the date.

3. Be punctual and consider the other persons nerves and feelings too.

4. Relax, take deep breaths and have an open stance. Do not fold your arms or stand with your legs crossed.

5. Actively listen. Respond specifically to the other person's conversation. Show sincere interest.

6. Ask open-ended questions such as How? and Why? and say, *"Tell me more about the music you like", "What kind of holidays do you enjoy the most?" "How did you feel when you retired?" "Why do you drive a Range Rover?"* Avoid closed questions that result in simple, *"Yes"* or *"No"* answers.

7. Have the attitude that you can make a new friend because if there are no sparks between you, a friendship can often lead to other connections and possibly *'the right one'*.

8. Look for common ground but be open minded about differences because you may find this person broadens your experiences and opens up new opportunities for you.

Be Open to Love

Of course, many women do genuinely fall in love and find a warm and lasting love. Being brave leads lots of mature women back into long lasting and loving relationships.

Mature lovers who are prepared to understand and be patient, can use their imagination with romantic gestures and be sensitive and tender can still arouse each other to enjoy sex. This can reignite sexual desire and bring the bedroom alive with intimacy between a couple and your sexual activity can change for the better because you decide together, how you want to it to be.

If you feel this is for you then *'older'* can mean *'bolder'* and you have plenty of advice here to keep you safe so go and have fun because a new adventure awaits you. You just need to take the first step and go out there. Join a dating site, take up a course or go on holiday. Let yourself grow slowly and do not expect too much at first because you may not find love straight away.
Take your time, there are lots of lovely enriching experiences for you to enjoy and trust yourself to attract the right person into your heart because that person is looking for you too and you both deserve a lasting love.

The most common issue for women involves their appearance and feeling unattractive. In a recent interview, actress, writer and activist,

Emma Thompson has stated that in her view, *"...women are brainwashed from very early on to disapprove, and to not see things in the mirror that they can accept."*

It is often difficult for mature women to believe they are attractive and desirable just as they are so, being brave is the key to moving forward. Once a mutual attraction is recognised, mature lovers are unlikely to place appearance as their main priority for wanting to be with someone and both men and women are more interested in how they make each other feel emotionally. They both want to feel wanted, excited and satisfied and when there is love as well then they can create a lasting relationship.

You may begin a relationship with low self-esteem and lack confidence about your ability to interest a lover and keep a partner satisfied but many of my clients say that having met someone special, they are relaxed and comfortable and they are having the best sex they have ever had and you can expect the same.

Nature is looking after you. When you fall in love with someone later in life it can be bonding and create a sincere devotion in a way that may not have been in younger relationships. This is so that you are both kept safe, feel valued and are both cared for in this stage of life. Later relationships are often more loving, kinder and more meaningful for both partners. In the same way, many couples in long standing relationships who have spent their lives together also find their later relationship is the most relaxed and happiest phase of their lives.

Ultimately, age does not have to be a problem in relationships or the bedroom and you can both have a wonderfully intimate time based on your mutual desire to nurture each other and to feel appreciated and valued together. When it comes to falling in love and finding yourself a nurturing, sexually satisfying and happy relationship, it is totally possible. You CAN fall in love with a kind and stable partner and find someone that suits you to share your life with so that you CAN have a happy and fulfilling relationship.

Women Welcome Wealth

Wanting More

A few women organise pension plans early in life but most have a precarious working life and are still frequently disappointed in the provision they have made. There does come a point when you cannot avoid the question of your future after retirement and this awareness may develop as a slow realisation or as a sudden flash of recognition. Whichever it is the time arrives when you must work out the practicalities of your financial situation for your *'Seenager years'*, your third age, your middle-age, your senior years or whatever you refer to it as. Sadly, for many women this comes too late in their lives and they worry that they may not have made enough provision for the longevity they expect.

You might be surprised how many women in the UK are over 60 years old are officially homeless because for various reasons they could not sustain their jobs and subsequently their mortgages or rent. In the UK many women fell into a pension gap and unable to secure further employment, they have had to wait until they turn 66/67 years old before they became eligible for their state pensions and any support they may have needed.

Thousands of women have been *'sofa surfing,'* staying with family and friends, living in campervans and house-sitting to provide a roof over their heads. If you are currently one of these women who did not have the understanding or the time to make extra provision for yourselves you may be in difficulty and chaos that leave you struggling with your mental health but you need to take good advice and not struggle alone. Ask for help and advice from groups such as the Citizens Advice Bureau, Age Concern and your local councils and your councillors.

Thinking Ahead

Here are 4 examples to demonstrate the type of lifestyle and financial situations that mature women are considering when they think about their eventual retirement. Obviously, there are many more variants than these but hopefully these make you think about your own situation if you are looking ahead or maybe have already reached your retirement years.

Do any of these resemble your own position?

1) **You have worked fulltime all your life** and either you alone or you and your partner have saved, invested and planned for your later years. You will probably be thinking about your state and private pensions and how you can capitalise on your wise decisions and perhaps you expect to have inheritances due from relatives so you probably feel you are in a good position for your retirement years.

2) **You have worked fulltime most of your life** and either you alone or you and your partner have a property and state and private pensions. You probably feel you are in a fair position for your retirement years. However, you may continue to work full time or possibly part time for as long as possible to avoid downgrading your lifestyle. You probably expect to eventually downsize your home but if you are lucky, you might have an expected inheritance from parents so you hope your retirement years will be comfortable.

3) **You have worked a mixture of part time and full time all your life** and either you alone or you and your partner have serious concerns about your retirement years. You may have a small amount of pension but you will need to continue part

time work for as many years as you are allowed to work by your employer. You expect to downgrade your lifestyle and your home and your retirement years are already unclear and you expect your future to remain uncertain.

4) **You have not worked at all during your life** for a variety of reasons and without any private pensions nor having paid any national insurance. Without any investments you alone or you and your partner dread your retirement years. You are anxious about downgrading your lifestyle and your home. You dislike thinking about your retirement years because you expect retirement to be very difficult for you.

Alternatively, it may be complicated and you have made adequate or excellent provision for yourself either alone or with a partner but have lost track of your private pension and have become confused about different pension schemes you once belonged to. Perhaps you are bereaved or divorcing or you may have cohabited with a partner for many years and have no legal rights to their home, their pensions or their financial assets.

Maybe you have disabilities or illnesses since planning your retirement or possibly you are one of the many women who have found themselves jobless and homeless in the last few years because of changes to the state pensionable age. Maybe for various reasons you retired from your job earlier than your state pension began and are finding it difficult or impossible to find well paid employment.

Employment and Leadership

For women who are in employment their pensions are only a part of the concerns about their future. Employment for many perimenopausal and menopausal women can become a challenging situation and many women say they need support to remain in their jobs because their symptoms are so debilitating. In the UK there is currently a drive for better work conditions for women during menopause and women are hopeful that initiatives will be embraced by employers.

For example, the Mayor of London's outline for change. Employers and society are realising that women make up half the population and half the workforce and it makes financial sense to keep women working because it is costly to lose so many hours and days to sick leave or to recruit when these women give up their jobs.

Many thousands of women currently leave their careers and leadership roles because they cannot cope with menopausal symptoms, medical appointments, procedures and long stressful working hours. They also feel pushed out because of lack of sympathetic managers and understanding of their condition.

This is not just about loss of employees but also a loss of valuable experience and expertise. It is also, financially costly to employers to recruit and fill their roles. The experience, training and skills are costly to replace and it causes upheaval within many companies and organisations. Nationally, it is poor economics to ignore such a large percentage of the workforce especially when women choose easier employment over their career or to work less hours or stop working altogether. It also means they spend less and their economic contribution is also lost. Many women are disadvantaged by losing career, income and pension opportunities whilst raising children and usually working part time for many years.

Women who leave their employment frequently find themselves needing financial support because they often lose their homes as they end up in lower paying jobs with less money. It is a spiral that involves deteriorating mental and physical health that can be avoided and the UK government is currently making HRT more easily available and more affordable and hopefully, free to women.

On International Women's Day 2022, the Mayor of London Sadiq Khan announced world-leading reforms to break what he referred to as the *'last taboo in the workplace'*. This is intended to stop discrimination and stigma and promote education and discussion around how women can be supported in their jobs. For example, employers are being asked to provide quiet rooms for women who need time out for extreme symptoms. This is to give menopausal symptoms the same recognition and respect as any other health issue.

A Brief Summary of Sadiq Khan's Policy

Employers are required to:

- Educate themselves and staff on menopause.

- Recognise the long term effects of the menopause.

- Accept thar staff experiencing menopause are entitled to request suitable support and workplace adjustments.

- Ensure that the working environment is comfortable wherever possible, for instance with temperature-controlled areas.

- Make flexible adjustment to the working day in order to accommodate the need to take breaks if symptoms become severe.

- Allow time off to attend medical appointments or make suitable changes to work tasks when experiencing symptoms.

- Ensure all staff are responsible for having a general awareness of menopause issues and to challenge inappropriate behaviour or derogatory remarks about the menopause.

The policy states that, *'This new approach also aims to challenge the taboo surrounding menopause, which can prevent staff from accessing the support they need or leave them feeling embarrassed or anxious in the workplace'*.

In particular, this policy asks employers to create a new working environment and culture in which staff can discuss their symptoms without stigma or discrimination. Employers are expected to educate themselves and their staff on the subject and also to support staff by being flexible so they can continue to be effective in their roles.

This is promising and I look forward to these changes becoming the *'norm'* nationwide and to more helpful initiatives in the future.

Business and Entrepreneurship

Many women who are in demanding physical roles or positions with intensive and heavy workloads look forward to working less as they grow older. They try to negotiate changes to their hours and the possibility of dropping days whereas others in more satisfying or lighter jobs look forward to continuing their employment and maintaining their status quo for as long as possible.

For those that choose to transform their careers or because of redundancy, need to reapply for their jobs, often need to attend interviews they find challenging. It can be years since they tried *'selling'* themselves to a new employer and many women who perceive their age to be a barrier to being considered for a new job see this process as an uphill struggle. If they are close to retirement age, they frequently feel stuck and find themselves unable to find new employment despite being willing and being capable. Some clients have told me they found the idea of retraining in a new job as well as possibly studying and sitting exams or maybe relocating as extremely daunting and stressful.

Also, menopause with its physical, mental and emotional changes frequently comes at a time when women are caring for parents and older relatives alongside young grandchildren. At the same time that they find themselves in these *'sandwich years'*, they are wondering if they have enough income in the years ahead and it is not surprising that many women say they believe their age stacks against them.

Yet these women also instinctively know they have the potential to pursue their own interests and to experience the freedom they have promised themselves if only they could find a way to achieve this.

One option that is attractive to growing numbers of ladies who are about to retire and already retired is to take the transferable skills from their industry or a hobby or a sport and create a business enterprise that suits their personal commitments better whilst also providing the income they want.

More and more women are choosing to develop more than one stream of income by establishing a wide range of investments, trading stocks, consultancies, agencies, coaching programmes, training companies or product sales, services, hosting exhibitions, seminars and retreats and more.

Senior Entrepreneurship amongst women has been steadily on the rise because they can be time rich and therefore be more available to take up any lucrative opportunities. This sudden increase in women of all ages starting businesses or becoming self-employed is largely because of the social changes brought about by *'work from home technology'* and the onset of 'remote working' is one of the effects of the pandemic lockdowns and many societies are shifting their values and priorities. This is an era of female empowerment, leadership and self-employment that none of us guessed would manifest so quickly and mature women are a large part of this new business landscape.

Women who are committed to their careers long term are doing better than they have for many years because leadership roles are more available to them now. However, clients tell me they are still being side-lined and they feel they can only have the lifestyle they desire and fulfil their full potential by working for themselves. This is why so many are taking phased or early retirement in pursuit of their happiness and health.

The emergence of so many successful women who are in the latter stage of their lives but are still productive and contributing their wealth of knowledge, experience and wisdom to society and the economy, is inspiring. The years ahead are likely to be the most creative and satisfying for middle aged ladies who want it all but on their own terms and in their own time. This next generation of senior women is the first to embrace ageing as a positive opportunity to achieve a working life that suits their female physical, mental and emotional wellbeing especially after menopause. You can also be part of these exciting times.

When choosing a suitable Financial Advisor

Be Realistic and Seek the Right Advice

Financial security may be on your mind and so it is useful to consider all of your income, your outgoings and your assets to understand what you are likely to have to live on in the years ahead.

- **Income** – from pensions, any inheritances, wages from employment or business income, investment interest and savings. – **Assess what your income is likely to be.**
- **Outgoings** – your mortgage or rent, household costs, vehicle costs, travel, insurances, clubs, care of any dependants and maintenance, debts. – **Work out what you are paying for and evaluate its value.**

- **Assets** – property, jewellery, art, vehicles, music rights, antiques. – **Consider what you own that could be sold.**

Once you have done this you can decide if the changes you want to make are sensible or not and it is good to request advice and support from a financial advisor.

Given that you are expected to live a long life you may well decide that you need more income and you may decide that alongside your employment or after retirement that you will start a business or become self-employed.

When assessing your financial future choose your advisor carefully and make sure they understand what you want to achieve in both the short term and the long term.

Do not assume they understand you. Check this with them. They need to be willing to sit with you and explain things in clear language to make sure that you understand. I do not wish to be patronising here or assume you are not intelligent but I have come across so many women who have made big mistakes through lack of confidence to assert themselves and ask questions when they have spoken to financial advisors. You need to understand exactly what you want and you need to understand the details of what they are proposing.

"... you can create an honourable livelihood, where you take your skills and use them and you earn a living from it, it gives you a sense of freedom and allows you to balance your life the way you want."

Dame Anita Roddick
Businesswoman and Environmentalist

Business Success Over 50

Senior Entrepreneurship is Growing Fast

Do you believe that you have spent your entire life so far, working just to reach the *'last stage'* of your life which involves physical decline, financial limitation and emotional sadness? Do you avoid thinking about it but you feel that every birthday is one step closer to a miserable old age?

Well, I believe it can be and should be, the most exciting time of your life in which you finally have time for self-discovery and reinvention so that you can continue into your latter years of your *'Third Age'* to live a fulfilling and happy life.

Also, like the majority of women over 50 years old in the UK you may expect that your income and lifestyle is likely to be cut considerably when you retire. The number of women with financial security for their retirement is lower than you might think and even if you have great retirement funds you still need to ask yourself how long that money will last and support your lifestyle when your current expected life-span is to live to an age over 100 years. As you are expected to have a long life, you will most likely want to look for one or more extra sources of income.

If the idea of being a businesswoman or being self-employed is new to you then you will also want to do some research and hopefully the following pages will inspire you to decide whether business IS for you or that business is NOT for you.

Assuming that when you first think about starting a business or being self-employed, even if its only part time, you are interested in creating more income then you need to make a plan. At times, you may doubt yourself and lack confidence to tackle what may seem like a huge change of mindset and skillset. However, it is all achievable if you take small steps forward and stay focused.

The first thing to do is to assess your skills, your talents and your passions. Evaluate the things you love to do and things you are good at and hopefully excel at. Also, consider the amount of time you have available to invest as well as how much money you have to start a business or to set up as self-employed. Remember that a business loan, government funding or charity funding may be possible for you if you wish to apply for one.

Next, do some more research into your ideas and talk to people running businesses in the sector you intend to open your business in. People in your own location may see you as a threat and be unhelpful. Therefore, it is best to contact people in other areas of the country and speak to people who will be honest and helpful.

You will then feel more confident about which type of business you might want. If you have no idea then contact me to help you find the best options for you to develop more income.

Decide what your business will be like and what will be best for your personal lifestyle. For example, how many hours will you work from home or in a shop or office and what will help you achieve your long term goals? It is important to think it all through.

What kind of business do you want? Who are customers and clients going to be and how will you find and attract them? Think about this and answer these questions. Remember these are examples to help you begin thinking about whether a business or self-employment are for you or if you are better suited to earning income through employment and other investments instead.

Do you want to …

* run a service based or product-based business?

* work alone?

* have a team working for you?

* have a business partnership?

* own a franchise business?

* a network marketing business?

* run a consultancy business?

* use your existing expertise or re-train?

* turn a hobby or a passion into business?

* work from home or find premises?

* hold and store stock?

* know what equipment, technology or staff you need?

* know how much initial outlay you will need?

I am sure you have thought of many more questions but these are a start and you will have a clearer image and idea of things you need to consider if you want to create the best business for you.

Keep in mind that business is similar in many ways to a job in that you have to put effort into it. Sometimes you progress through various jobs until you find one you love and sometimes you fall straight into the job of your dreams and business is similar. Take your time to find out what feels right for you and be open-minded because you may change your mind a couple of times.

If you have never been in business or been self-employed before then you have a lot to learn and having a mentor and coach to guide you, make sure you have a clear plan and lots of support in the early days prevents mistakes and wasting your precious time.

Although, you need to be happy in your business remember it is also about securing a good income for your future so that you can have a good lifestyle as well as a happy life.

"Know that you are worthy of love. Know that you are worthy of great things in life if you put your mind to it."

Alexandra Burke
Singer, Song Writer and Actress

~ Discovering You ~

What Is Coaching and Mentoring?

Coaching is not Counselling

Coaching is goal orientated and can quickly help you to assess the reality of a situation and set of circumstances and help you to work out your own solutions and subsequent strategies. You can then then take clear action to move forward at your own pace in your own way but with guidance and support and achieve the results and success you want.

Mentoring is not Coaching

Mentoring helps you to learn and be competent at a specific skill, process or strategy. Your mentor shares their own knowledge. skill and experience about a specific specialism and area of expertise with you. As you apply this fresh understanding you are then equipped to and replicate and build upon what they teach and share with you. This is often achieved in stages as and when you need the skills and knowledge and helps you to achieve your goals to a high level of success.

Blended Coaching and Mentoring

I use a blend of coaching with mentoring with clients and take you through a system starting with your physical, mental and emotional wellbeing and going through to discover and express your purpose and motivation. It is important to me that you are youthful, healthy and happy with the income and lifestyle you deserve.

"I've discovered this is your moment to reinvent yourself after years of focusing on the needs of everyone else. It's your opportunity to get clear about what matters to you and then to pursue that with all of your energy, time and talent."

Oprah Winfrey
TV Presenter, Producer, Actress and Author

Are You Ready?

Are you ready to REJUVENATE your life?

Are you ready to *Age Well* and *Live Well?*

Are you willing to TRANSFORM yourself?

Are you willing to *Feel Youthful* and *Look Younger?*

Are you able to CREATE your happiness?

Are you able to *Fulfil Your Dreams* and *Love Your Life?*

Be a *'Seenager'*

youthful, healthy and happy
with the income security you want

"It was like talking to a friend. She made it easy and helped me by knowing what I was trying to say.

Thank you, Victoria, for the guidance and support you have given me. I feel I can move forward now in all areas with confidence."

Jennifer Connelly
Fertility Reflexologist

Rejuvenation & Lifestyle Coaching

I offer a choice between these 3 programmes to help you relax, replenish and rejuvenate yourself and your life.

Be Calm, Be Resilient

3 Sessions - including access to supportive, informative and friendly on-line group. These sessions focus on your personal needs to help you to be clear about your way forward. These sessions are useful and for simple situations and making and quick progress.

Be Happy, Be Amazing

6 sessions - including access to a client only on-line group. Email and text support during the programme.

1 Free Bonus session to be taken at any time within 1 year period. these sessions focus on helping you to overcome your limitations to create your future happiness.

Further continuation programme – another 6 sessions to give you extended coaching and a deeper dive into your creativity and manifesting your best life, according to your personal needs or preferences.

Your sessions are following a structured 3 stage programme but give you a bespoke service, tailored to your specific needs,

These sessions help you to expand your vision for yourself and achieve more than you realise for yourself. It gives you more in depth understanding of what you want and how to achieve it.

Rejuvenate your physical and emotional as well as your psychological wellbeing and mind set.

1. I show you how to use simple techniques and exercises with support-sheets so that you can deep dive into your lifestyle to transform your feelings and your energy. This means you have a calm mind to make clear choices.
2. Knowing what you want in your life and what matters to you helps you to move forward with focused enthusiasm.
3. The programme is structured in 3 stages but the sessions are holistic and flexible, according to your individual needs.
4. Your wellbeing is a priority together we begin by focussing on increasing your resilience to stress and increasing your overall happiness.
5. Using various techniques that are appropriate for each stage of your *'journey'* I refer to both current science and research. With an understanding of neurology, psychology I take into consideration any spiritual, religious and philosophical approaches to the world.
6. I help you develop 4 core aspects of yourself so that you are rejuvenated in ways that are satisfying and empowering.

Your First Step to Clarity

Free 30mins Discussion
Plus a **Free E-book Guide** *'Unstress Your Yourself'.*

If you would like to speak to me about rejuvenating yourself, your life and your purpose then you will find my details at the back of this book and I am happy for you to contact me now.

victoria@victoriasheridancoach.com

Business Coaching

If you are already an entrepreneur or if you decide to become self-employed or to establish a business of your own, then I also offer coaching programmes designed specifically to help you develop the best skills and practices that can create the income and work-life balance you want.

~ Make it in Business ~

3 sessions with online support group.

~ Make the Business You Want ~

6 sessions with client only online support group. Email and text support during the programme.

Free Bonus session to be taken at any time within 1 year period.

The all sessions are bespoke and tailored to your individual type of business or enterprise.

Your personal dreams, goals; create a great strategy for profit and success and focus on the strategies you need to fulfil your plans. Achieve your purpose and the outcomes that you want.

You decide which programme is best suited to you before starting and sessions are undertaken at times according to the pace your specific project.

1. I take you from start to finish in your business plan and show you how to use simple exercises and support-sheets to plan and complete your quickest and effective steps forward.
2. Using support-sheets, I guide you to focus your mindset and your mental approach, so that you can have clarity to make clear decisions based on your values and vision.
3. Knowing what your goals and priorities are and what is important to you, you choose the strategies you need for your business development.
4. Sessions are delivered in accordance with your particular business plan, but within the overall programme structure.
5. Your success is a priority by transforming your weaknesses and developing your strengths to help you build a profitable enterprise that also makes you happy.

~ Your First Step to Clarity ~

Free 30mins Discussion
Plus a **Free E-book Guide** *'Business Success'*.

If you would like to speak to me about starting a business or expanding an existing one to suit your goals then I am happy for you to contact me now.

victoria@victoriasheridancoach.com

Inspirational Reading

These books that have influenced me and my clients.
I trust you enjoy them too.

Maya **Angelou**, (1969), *The Caged Birds Sings*, Random House.
Sarah Ban **Breathnach**, (1997), *Simple Abundance*, Bantam.
Jan **Brown**, (2019) *Learn Reiki,* Janet Brown.
Julia **Cameron**, (2016), *The Artist's Way*, Macmillan.
Jean **Carper**, (1997), *Stop Ageing Now,* Thorsons.
Deepak **Chopra**, (2001), *Grow Younger, Live Longer*, Rider.
HH **Dalai** Lama, (2000), *Ancient Wisdom, Modern World*, New Ed edition Abacus Press.
Wayne **Dyer**, (1998), *Wisdom of the Ages,* Thorsons.
Jenny **Eclair**, (2020), *Older and Wider; A Survivor's Guide to the Menopause,* Quercus Editions Ltd.
Hilary **Ellis,** (2020) *A Personal Philosophy: Your Truth, My Truth, A Journey to Peace,* Hilary Ellis.
Liz **Earle**, (2016), *Healthy Menopause*, Orion.
Mariella **Frostrup** & Alice Smellie, (2022) *Cracking the Menopause*, Bluebird.
Lyn **Hardy**, (2021) *The Aging Games: How to Come Out a Winner*, Independent.
Louise **Hay**, (1984), *You Can Heal Your Life*, Hay House.
Rosanna **Ienco**, (2009) *Awakening the Divine Soul: Finding Your Life's Purpose,* O Books.
Wendy **Jennings,** (2020) *From Cancer to Coddiwomple – A Story of Love and Daring to Dream,* Coddiwomple Publishing.
Genny **Jones**, (2016) *Crown of Smiles*, 1st Edition, Mindset Makeover Mission Publishing.
Helen **Keller,** (1991), *The Story of My Life,* Bantam Classic.
Phillip **McGraw**, (2001), *Self-Matters,* Simon and Shuster.
Louise **Newson**, (2019), Menopause; Manual, Haynes.
Christiane **Northrup**, (2015), *Goddesses Never Age*, Hay House.

Florence Scovel **Shinn**, (2016), *The Game of Life and How to Play It,* Hay House.
David A. **Sinclair**, (2019), *Life Span*, Thorsons.
Delia **Smith,** (2022) You Matter: The Human Solution, Mensch Publishing.
Donna **Still,** (2019) *The Essence of Being: Poetry on the Nature of Life,* Donna Still.
Eckart **Tolle**, (1997), *The Power of Now,* New World.
David **Weeks,** (1998), *Superyoung*, Hodder & Stoughton.

~ Other Support ~

Guest Contributors

Additional Support For You

Rejuvenating your life and becoming a *'Seenager'* is a very personal and experience and needs to consider your individual needs and unique lifestyle.

There are other aspects of life that you want to improve as part of the *'refreshingly new you'* that you want to become and the most common ones are -

- Restyling your personal appearance.
- Securing sound financial advice.
- Maintaining the strength of your pelvic floor.

As you rejuvenate yourself and your life, you may want more specific information and advice, on these particular aspects. Therefore, it is my pleasure to introduce you to three professional women who have kindly, contributed their professional insights to the next three chapters.

Sarah Grant is an award-winning Independent Image and Style Consultant, Alison Wright is also an award-winning Personal Financial Adviser, Julie Bartlett is a double award-winning Holistic Core Restore Coach.

Image Confidence

Lasting Impressions

by Sarah Grant

The woman who wears the wrong colour and style *disappears*

The woman who wears the right colour and style APPEARS

What does self-image mean to you?

Why is it important?

Self-image is a mental picture of how we see ourselves physically, but also emotionally and psychologically. I am going to share with you tips and information on how to find your *unique*, positive self-image. In life, we only have 7 seconds to make a good first impression, especially for that all-important job, going on a new date or any occasion where you are meeting people for the first time. Did you know that 80% of our communication is visual and only 20% is the spoken word? When we wear our *unique colours and style,* our confidence and self-esteem are boosted. Knowing that you look and feel good, allows you to present the best you. We have all been in situations where our confidence has been knocked. It may have been through a divorce, job loss, bereavement, menopause, weight gain, illness, or any other life crisis we may have experienced. As women, we deserve to make the best of ourselves, but we often spend our lives putting others needs before our own. Now is the time to put yourself first. Dress how you want to feel not how you feel.

You know you are worth it.

COLOUR

Do you wear a lot of black?

Ask yourself; why do you wear a lot of black?

Colour affects our emotions in many ways. It can evoke memories from a previous experience. Ladies frequently say to me that navy blue or bottle green reminds them of their school uniform and as they had to endure the uniform for so many years, they have never worn those colours again.

However, changing the colours you wear, to suit your individual *unique colouring,* can also, have a positive effect on your emotions. The colours you wear benefit you, not just by the way you look, but also by the way you feel.

The benefits of wearing your unique colours are -

1. Improves overall appearance.
2. Skin looks clearer.
3. Eyes look clearer.
4. Enhances levels of confidence and self-esteem.
5. Receives a positive response from people.
6. Creates a totally coordinated wardrobe.
7. Make choosing clothes much easier.
8. Saves money.
9. Saves time.
10. Gives better value from purchases.
11. Ensures all your clothes are worn.

Have you ever worn an outfit and someone has said to you, "*Wow! you look amazing.*" It is often because you are wearing one of your *unique colours and/or style.* I have a coat that I have nicknamed my '*Magic Coat.*' I can guarantee that every time I wear it, I get compliments. This coat is my best *unique colour*, coral. I feel like a million dollars in this coat and it adds sunshine to my day even when it is wet and dreary.

People usually wear black because they want to blend into the background, they think it makes them appear slimmer or they do not know what colours suit them. I know that I look like a ghost if I was to wear black and it makes the lines on my face appear deeper and that is something I certainly do not want. If it is one of your colours then that is fine but as we get older our skin tone changes and skin becomes transparent and black can make us look much older than we really are.

We tend to mirror our environment with our clothes. For example, in winter, women will turn towards dark colours and alternatively, to brighter colours in summer. I know we are often governed by what is in the shops at any given season but colour can be added to our winter clothes by wearing a scarf with our '*Unique Colours.*'

Knowing my own colour direction, which for me is *Light* and *Warm,* during the winter it can sometimes be difficult to find these colours what I do to overcome this is to buy my jumpers during the summer and pair them with long sleeved thermal tops underneath. Look for shops that sell colourful light-weight thermals with a variety of necklines and sleeve lengths in several colours to cover all bases.

A Colour Analysis determines your *unique colours* and is based on your individual skin tone, eye colour and natural hair colour.

At home you can remove your make-up stand in front of a mirror and place a large piece of black fabric or clothing across the top half of your body/neck. Look to see if it leaves a dark shadow under your chin and the effect it has on your skin and lines. Next, do the same with navy blue or grey. Which one looks best against your complexion?

You can play with all the colours to find out if you are a warm or cool complexion and whether you should wear light or bright colours. Always remember your eye is drawn to the lightest and brightest colour.

BODY SHAPE

What shape are you?

You may be confused about what body shape you are because it has to do with proportions of your body and you need a professional to assess you in terms of styling.

The benefits of knowing your body shape are -

1- Creates positive first impressions.
2- Choices of clothes are perfect and comfortable.
3- Makes shopping much easier.
4- Boosts confidence and self-esteem.
5- Saves you money.
6- Saves time.

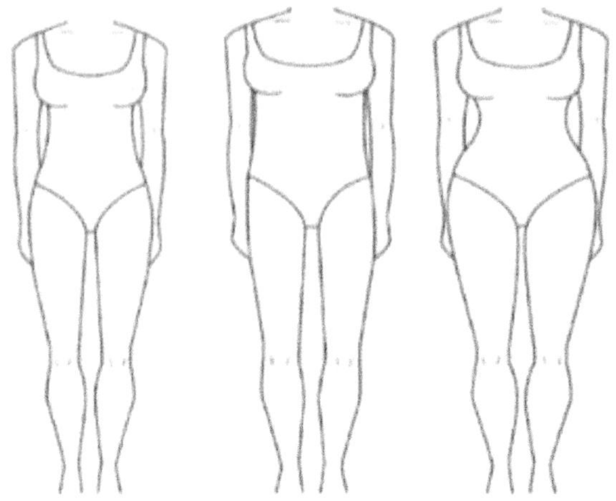

Most people think of body shapes as Pear, Apple or Hourglass but I work with three body shapes. Straight, Semi-shaped and Shaped and I relate to your silhouette, the sides of your body.

STRAIGHT: The body line will not have a defined waist and they tend to put weight on around the tummy area. They usually have great legs and appear longer and as their shoulders may be wider than their hips, they can be top heavy.

SEMI-STRAIGHT: The body line will have a slightly defined waist and they tend to put their weight on evenly balanced and they are often the easiest to dress if slim.

SHAPED: The body line has a very defined waist and they will carry their weight around their hips and bottom which appears to shorten the leg. They may have wider hips than shoulders.

To assess your shape, all other aspects are considered such as the width of your shoulders, arm length, hem line, neckline, and face shape. Your bust line and the length of your body are also considered. As we mature our bodies change. Your fundamental shape stays the same but your waist thickens and this is the area most women want to disguise. When you know which areas of your body you want to emphasise and which ones to conceal. You learn how to balance your body to give you the best look.

WARDROBE PERSONALITY/STYLE

What is your wardrobe personality/style?

The benefits of knowing your personal wardrobe/style personality are -

1. Understanding why you choose certain garments or accessories.
2. Prevents you from making impulse buys.
3. Helps to identify shops and brands that sell your style.
4. Boosts your confidence and self-esteem.
5. Creates a coordinated wardrobe that works for any occasion.
6. Saves time.
7. Saves money.

Think about the impression you want to make in any given situation. Part of having an image and styling consultation with me would include you completing a useful questionnaire which helps me to determine your wardrobe personality and style.

WARDROBE PERSONALITIES

There are 5 Wardrobe Personalities but you usually have one predominant personality, which has a strong influence and a couple of the other types with weaker influence. When you find your *unique personality*, it helps you to understand why you want to look and feel a certain way. Shopping becomes easier and you will start to recognise the shops and make of clothing that suits your personality best.

The 5 wardrobe personalities are -

DRAMATIC: They have a big personality and love to make an entrance, appear confident and are hard to ignore. They like to show their individuality not just through their clothes but also their hair style and accessories which are big and bold. They like to explore the latest trends and they are more likely to spend a lot on a statement item and less on their basics.

NATURAL: They are relaxed and often feel comfortable within themselves. They like easy to wear clothes that allow them freedom to move easily and natural fabrics. They do not like shopping and will struggle if they have a special event to go to as they do not know where to go as far as shopping is concerned. They do not wear make-up unless they must and their hair will be simple and easy to style.

CLASSIC: They appear elegant, in control and organised as their clothes are simple, well-cut, and timeless. They find dressing down difficult. Their favourite colours are usually their best neutrals and they prefer natural fabrics. Shoes and handbags will be of decent quality but they tend to gravitate to more expensive items, however, they purchase less often, as value is important to them. Jeans can be a struggle for them but they frequently team them with classic shirts and jackets.

GAMINE: *('gam' as in glamour, 'mine' as in sheen)* They tend to have a *'sporty'* personality and a have fun element to their choices. They are classic dressers but with a quirky side to them. They like jeans with maybe a bit of detail on the pocket or a jacket with detail on the shoulders. Shoes tend to be trainers or a simple shoe or sandal and they like to use some colour with their neutral colours. They tend to be neat and tidy with hairstyles simple, chic, and easy to do with minimal make-up to give a soft look.

ROMANTIC: They love to express themselves through their clothes as they are feminine and are often creative. They are tactile and love the texture of different fabrics such as lace, velvet, chiffon, and silk. Their clothes will usually have embellishment on them. They like to present themselves looking their best on all occasions. Hair and make-up are important and generally will not leave the house without it.

I hope this has given you food for thought about your individual style and has inspired you to explore who you are. Working with a Personal Stylist will help you to determine your unique wardrobe/style and personality.

UNDERWEAR

It is vital to get the correct underwear but 80% of ladies wear the incorrect bra size *(UK)*. This is usually because the bra is too big around the back and the cup is too small. I used to buy a 34C *(UK)* but when measured correctly I was a size 32E *(UK)* so I recommend going to a bra specialist as they know their products so well.

Panties with no visible panty line (VPL) are the best to wear under a tight-fitting dress or pair of trousers but always be aware that lace will show through light weight fabric. All-in-one body shapers are fabulous to give you that smooth look and there are so many out there it is worth trying a few.

MAKE-UP

How do you feel when you wear make-up?

The benefits of wearing the most suitable make-up are –

1. Boosts Confidence and self-esteem.
2. Creates a good first impression.
3. Evens out skin tone and covers blemishes.
4. Brightens and wakes you up.
5. Creates a youthful effect.
6. Saves money.

Make-up should enhance us not dominate us. As we mature our skin loses its elasticity, it becomes thinner, more transparent, and fragile. We should take care of our skin. Exposure to the sun is responsible for most of the visible ageing.

I am 60 years old, *"I like to say 60 years young"*. I always clean, tone and moisturise every night and every morning. I exfoliate once or twice a week and use rehydrating face mask once a week.

Our skin needs hydration and drinking water is the one of the best ways rehydrate it. Try to drink 1 to 2 litres of water a day as this will also improve the appearance of our skin, energy, sleep and helps aid weight loss. I took part in a Facebook challenge, which was to drink 2 litres of water a day for a month. The difference in my skin was incredible, it was more hydrated, I had more energy and I sleep was much improved. I must admit I do not always get my 2 litres a day. My daughter did the challenge and commented how her skin was far less dry.

Many women tell me that they do not know how to apply make-up. They are stuck in their old routine and do not know which foundation to buy as there are so many available.

A tip for buying the correct foundation is to put a small amount on the jawline and gently rub it in, if you cannot see it, it is the correct colour, if you can see it, then it is the wrong colour. It can be very confusing when you are shopping for foundation so, I would advise that you ask the assistant to match it up with your skin tone and then request a sample to take home with you and try in natural lighting, as the lighting in shops, gives you a false indication.

As we mature, many of us find our eye lids can become heavy and some of us can lose the definition of the eye socket. I show my clients that by using eye shadow the correct way they can give the illusion of lifting their eye lids and opening-up their eyes.

INSIGHTFUL EXPERIENCES.

One day, my neighbour came out of her drive and we chatted. I said to her *"You look amazing where are you going?"* Telling me only the name of a shop, she then proceeded to tell me about her son who was *'going travelling'*. and had requested a work permit for New Zealand, all of which made her feel very down. However, she had made the decision that she did not want to feel like that, so she had put on make-up and a beautiful top with a lovely skirt, to lift her spirits and she felt better. This shows how, having a positive mindset on how we dress, can boost our confidence. and self-esteem when we are feeling down. She also had a huge smile and our smile is one of our best assets, because it opens us up, makes us feel good and shows people that we are happy to see them.

I also worked with a lady who would not wear trousers. When I asked why, she said, *"My father told me I had a big bottom when I was a little girl."* I found it so sad she had lived her life believing this. I asked her if she would try a pair of trousers on which she did. They were the correct colour and shape for her unique style, when she looked in the mirror, she loved them and said, *"My bottom doesn't look big."*

To help her understand her difficulty with her self-image, I took her through a Timeline 5 exercise. The exercise helped her to remove the limiting beliefs about her shape that she had held on to for so long. About five weeks later I phoned her to see how she was getting on with the clothes she had purchased and she confirmed that she loved everything she had bought.

My final question to her was '*Do you wear trousers?"* she replied, *"All the time."*

When you buy clothes, you must '*Love'* them because if you do not you simply will not wear them. You should love even your basic top, I always buy good quality basic T-shirts with a low neckline, as I have a fuller bust and I know they will always look good.

A client will sometimes ask me, what do you think of this top on me? And I always reply to her that it is her choice and as she is the one wearing it and she must make the decision. I guide my clients through the process and say to them, *"Imagine your wardrobe is in front of you, put the top/dress in it and close the door. Wait a minute, now open it and do you still choose to put it on."* This never fails to give them the answer.

Sarah Grant is an award-winning expert in her field as an Image Consultant and NLP Practitioner. She supports and encourages women to be the best possible version of themselves from the inside to the outside. **www.sarahjanegrant.co.uk**

Financial Confidence

All names of clients have been changed for privacy and confidentiality purposes.

Your Income Matters

by Alison Wright

As women are now fully empowered and can make their own financial decisions, this means that we can take control and ownership of our money and decide what it means and, importantly what it is able do for all of us.

Having robust financial plans, even if these start from very modest beginnings, can help you to have clarity, direction and relief from worry. The opposite of this is that an inadequate or non-existent financial strategy which can potentially lead to you to more stress, anxiety, lack of sleep and other health issues.

A 2017 report for the Money and Mental Health Policy Institute, called *'Seeing through the Fog'*, examined the way that depression affects our ability to manage our money. It highlighted that people with depression, struggle to deal with the complexity of money matters, because the condition impairs *'focus'* and *'working memory'*. It also affects our ability to plan and make decisions and it damages our *'psychomotor functioning'*, so that routine tasks become arduous and insurmountable.

Seeking professional help to make wise decisions about your money and income is more popular than ever especially amongst women and you are most likely to seek personal financial advice when you experience a life event. These include, paying for a divorce, birth of a child or grandchild, dealing with redundancy and coping with ill health or bereavement. However, you are also likely to seek advice if you decide to buy a home, send your children off to university, plan for your retirement or want to invest an inheritance.

To help you recognise some of the possible scenarios that you may find yourself in, here are some of my case studies. These are indicative of some of the issues clients that I have worked with over the years have encountered, but in each case, the names and some of the details, have been changed for confidentiality purposes.

Client A: Rachel

A few years ago, I met with a new client called Rachel. At 34 years old Rachel had recently separated from her husband after 6 years of marriage and had a young son of 4 years of age that she was caring for.

Rachel had taken a career break from her job as a PA for a London based Construction Company, to raise her son, whilst her husband continued with his well-paid IT job. Reconciliation was not an option for Rachel and her husband and they had agreed to divorce, sell the family home and start afresh. Rachel was the daughter of close friends of some existing clients of mine and she was introduced to me for an initial chat because she had no idea how to begin organising her finances and preparing for the future.

Quite frankly, Rachel was in shock, shaken by the sudden breakdown of her marriage, on the grounds of her husband's infidelity and did not know which way to turn first. However, Rachel knew that she needed to get her financial arrangements in order that she could plan ahead for her and her son but she did not know how to go about it, or where to start.

The divorce proceedings were underway and agreements had already been made about child maintenance and the division of assets including the share of the family home. Fortunately, this left her with enough money to put down a sizeable deposit on a new, albeit modest home, for her and her son. Rachel had also decided to go back to work and had secured a job with a local family firm as an administrator which allowed her to manage her hours around her son's schooling.

Our initial discussions covered:

- A new monthly budget of incomings and outgoings.
- Establishing a new Will.
- Requirement for a mortgage to assist the purchase of her new home.
- Review of her income tax position.
- Getting a state pension forecast (Form BR19 www.gov.uk).
- Looking at her existing pensions with current and former employers.
- Reviewing her savings and those of her Son (e.g., Child Trust Fund/Junior ISA).
- Life and Critical Illness Cover and protection against her being unable to work due to ill health.

Rachel had postponed taking the previous pension that she arranged with her former employer and this remained deferred whilst she had fresh Workplace Pension in place with her new employer. It was time to assess whether she was also entitled to any of her ex-husband's pension as part of her divorce. This pension sharing order, if agreed between her and her husband, could be part of the final financial settlement and a valuable contribution towards her own retirement planning.

Clearly, there was a lot for us to discuss, so the first step was for me to help Rachel establish her priorities and to tackle each of these items in order. Understandably, her main priority was to secure finance for her new home and to ensure that adequate life and sickness cover was in place to cover, not only the mortgage, but also to secure additional funds to look after her son if she passed away or became seriously ill up till the point he was no longer financially dependent.

When you are looking at both mortgages and life/sickness cover, it is advisable to seek advice from a professional like me who can access the whole of the market and all that is available so that the best products are researched thoroughly to ensure that your needs and budget are met. Therefore, we completed a comprehensive Budget Plan for Rachel to confirm that she could manage her monthly commitments for mortgage, utilities, childcare, food and fuel as well as making sure there was a little over for some fun.

It was also especially important that she was receiving the correct amount of net income and making full use of her tax allowances. I reviewed her personal taxation which was especially important at this time as Rachel made the transition from being a *'stay at home'* mum to becoming employed again.

Rachel became less concerned as she realised there were answers to her confusion and so, the next priority was to arrange for her to have a professionally drafted Will. This helped her to decide and direct what will happen to her Estate in the event of her death. Rachel found this quite difficult as she needed to nominate Guardians to look after her son and Trustees to manage his finances until he became an adult. This *'age of majority'* is usually 18 years of age. I also carried out a full pension review for Rachel as this did not require any additional funding and I ascertained the status of her 'frozen' pension that was with her former employer. I discovered how much it was worth and how it was managed. By organising a State Pension forecast for Rachel, we were also able to see what she might need to do to make up any shortfall and to ensure that she receives the maximum State Retirement Pension that she will be entitled to at her State Retirement Age.

In figures obtained by the Pensions Review Service, it was estimated that in 2015, £2 billion was sitting unclaimed in UK frozen pension schemes! Several years on from this, the figure is likely to be higher!

Research undertaken by Age UK in 2013, found that 23% of British adults have at least one pension that they have lost track of and are therefore, failing to claim and receive benefits from these. Sometimes, but not always, it can be beneficial to transfer old pension arrangements to a new provider. For Rachel it meant that her pensions can potentially continue to increase in value, boost her retirement pot, all the while benefiting from ongoing advice. However, Rachel needed to consider the impact of other costs that could be involved in a transaction like this and I discussed this fully with her and gave her the advice she needed for her to make a clear and informed decision that she was comfortable with.

We should all be looking at our pension history and see if we have any plans from former employers, or personal arrangements taken out ages ago that we are no longer funding and to see if they are still giving us the most favourable financial outcomes. At the very least, a review like this can give you a clear and up to date understanding of what you have, where it is, what it is worth and what it is projected to provide when you retire.

Returning to Rachel; a full year after our first meeting, I helped her to review her savings proposition. She wanted to get fully settled in her new job and home and be confident that she could do more than just make ends meet. Rachel was doing well, loved her job and had gained a pay rise, had turned her house into a proper home for her and her son. She had even managed a short break away for them both during the school holidays. Rachel felt confident that she could set aside an amount every month to start some regular savings and we agreed to split the amount she had chosen between a cash-based savings account, that would provide her with a valuable buffer and a contribution into a regular savings stocks and shares Individual Savings Account (ISA).

The ISA should be held over the medium to longer term (5-15 years) to allow for capital growth and for the ups and downs of the markets. Before committing to the stocks and shares ISA we had a full and detailed discussion about the full nature of this type of investment and the associated risks and costs. If you are considering this type of investment or savings scheme, make sure you also, take advice on the risks and costs involved. It must be remembered that the value of an investment such as this can go down as well as up and past performance is no guide to future.

I have continued to see Rachel on a regular basis, at least once a year and we use our meeting time to review the plans she has put in place which include the regular savings ISA and her previous pension that we transferred over from her ex-employer. These reviews are essential to monitor the progress and performance of Rachel's plans and to make sure they remain on track and relevant for her goals, dreams and aspirations. The reviews also help Rachel to take into consideration any changes in her circumstances and I can inform her of any changes to Government legislation or changing conditions in the financial market that may influence our planning. Ultimately, this means that I can assess the situation and advise Rachel if she needs to take any action and when and if she might need to make any changes to help her to keep her financial planning secure. As her advisor, I feel it is important that Rachel feels empowered and not overwhelmed by my expertise.

Clients B: Keith and Pauline

I would now like to introduce you to Keith and Pauline, whom I met at a pre-retirement seminar where I was presenting a few years ago. Keith was planning on taking retirement. at the age of 60 which is five years earlier than originally planned but he felt that early retirement would suit both him and Pauline now that they had a couple of young grandchildren and they wanted to spend more time with them and make good use of their prized motorhome and generally to travel more widely.

The purpose of the pre-retirement seminar was to advise people of their various options at retirement and to give some general guidance regarding the range of choices available, including how to access income and how to manage their retirement fund in a tax efficient manner. Following the seminar itself, I arranged to go and meet them in their own home so that we could have a further discussion about what might be the best course of action for them and to have a look at whether Keith's Company Pension provided by his Employer would provide enough income for them both and be able to provide them with a comfortable retirement, despite the earlier retirement date.

Keith was fortunate to be a member of a Final Salary (Defined Benefit) Scheme and had worked for the same Company for 35 years. This is becoming less common nowadays as people are much more transient in their careers. During these conversations, we established that, alongside Keith's final salary pension scheme from his employer and the tax-free sum he would get upon taking retirement benefits they had also built up some significant savings by putting away surplus income over the last 8 to 10 years of their working lives particularly after their son and daughter left home and stopped being financially dependent on them. We established that it would be possible to generate some additional income from Keith's tax-free lump sum payable when his work pension commenced payment by making use of appropriate investment vehicles.

Additionally, Keith and Pauline agreed to designate some of their accumulated saving's capital to other investment options. This meant that we would be able to create a further income stream from their investments to supplement Keith's pension income. Furthermore, it meant that Pauline could afford to give up her part time job as a classroom. assistant so that they could both on embark on retirement together.

When considering how much savings capital we could use for more structured investments to help them meet their income goals we did have to be mindful to leave adequate levels of accessible cash in easy access accounts so that they had available funds for any short term, larger expenses as well as for emergencies.

Alongside establishing some tax efficient investments to provide them with an additional income stream we also looked at ways in which they could invest for their grandchildren and build up modest investment accounts for them that would allow them access once they reached the age of 18. Keith and Pauline felt that this could give each of them a valuable start in life by helping them in areas such as some of the costs of a university education or putting down a small deposit on a property. They were both keen to make a difference to their grandchildren while they were still alive so that they could see the benefits such a financial gift could make to the younger members of their family.

In assessing the overall tax position for Keith and Pauline, we looked at ways in which we could mitigate the liability to Inheritance Tax on their estate and discussed the various rates and allowances that are currently applicable and available to them. It is important to understand that any such planning needs reviewing on a regular basis as, not only might legislation change but of course there will be updates and alterations in their own situation and value of their assets, that will need to be accommodated in order to keep tax planning appropriate.

As with Rachel, I carried out ongoing regular reviews with Keith and Pauline to make sure their retirement plans remain on track and consistently meet their needs and wishes. These reviews will ensure that they always have enough funds to continue enjoying their life in the way that they wish. This included monitoring the growth of their investment portfolio and managing the risk. Also, ensuring that it could keep pace with inflation and maintain its value in real terms all the while generating income for them.

As well as the investment, income and tax planning I carried out for them, I also made sure that Keith and Pauline's Wills were up-to-date and accurately reflected their wishes. They were also advised to take out Power of Attorney so that trusted people could take over their financial affairs in the event of them losing capacity. In Keith and Pauline's case, they nominated each other and their two children to act as attorneys thereby ensuring that their financial affairs could be continued in the way that they would wish to themselves in the event of them being unable to act in their own right perhaps through dementia or as a result of a debilitating accident.

You hope that you never need to make use of the Powers of Attorney but in case you do, it is invaluable. As a direct result of a successful relationship with Keith and Pauline I was also introduced to their son and daughter and I went on to assist them with their own retirement and savings planning.

Client C: Emma

The final client I would like to introduce you to is Emma, a 74 year old lady, who had been a client of mine for several years but my most recent interaction with her was when her husband of 49 years passed away after a short illness. At the first meeting following her husband Bob's passing both her son and daughter were present to offer moral support and to satisfy themselves that their mother was getting appropriate advice. The main areas of concern for Emma were to ensure that she would have enough income to meet her regular outgoings and enough capital to be able to pay for any larger expenses. She also felty strongly as that she would like to be able to leave something behind for her family by way of an inheritance.

After Bob's death his former work pension was reduced by 50% under the spouse's benefit conditions, (other schemes may operate under different terms) and Emma's own State Retirement Pension was increased slightly. However, the household net income was only down by about 30% and Emma was understandably concerned.

During my time working with both Emma and Bob in the past, we had already established a number of investments for them and we decided, with the consent of her children, to rearrange some of these to provide her with some additional income and add some additional capital to boost the level of income that was able to be generated. Following the Probate process, we also added some of Bob's former holdings to Emma's cash accounts for valuable accessibility and security as well as making use of some of the offerings available via National Savings & Investments.

Emma had been reassured that her income and accessible cash needs were well catered for, therefore, she decided to gift some money to each of her 2 children now and this was used in each case to reduce their mortgage. This gifting was also part of the Inheritance Tax mitigation strategy that formed part of our discussions.

As with all my clients, I meet with Emma and her family regularly to ensure that she remains in control of her finances and that her standard of living can be maintained. During one of our more recent meetings, Emma delighted in telling me that she had treated the entire family to a holiday.

Throughout this chapter I have tried to encourage you not to let your financial situation cause you anxiety or to be overwhelmed by it all. I hope these case studies have given you some insights and my closing advice is that it is essential to seek help, guidance and advice to assist with your financial wellbeing as soon as possible. Make sure that the adviser you engage to work with you offers you clear, concise, tailored, honest and transparent advice and that your planning is reviewed as regularly as you renew your home insurance or service your car.

Being empowered to make the right financial decisions for you can enrich your life and provide may more choices, options and freedom to live the life you choose.

Alison Wright is a Personal Financial Adviser with over 30 years' experience, during which she has won several awards for building long-term, trusted relationships with clients by offering high standards of service and making the processes simple to eliminate stress. **www.alisonwright.co.uk**

Physical Confidence

Eliminate Embarrassment

by Julie Bartlett

My body, My Pelvic Floor and More

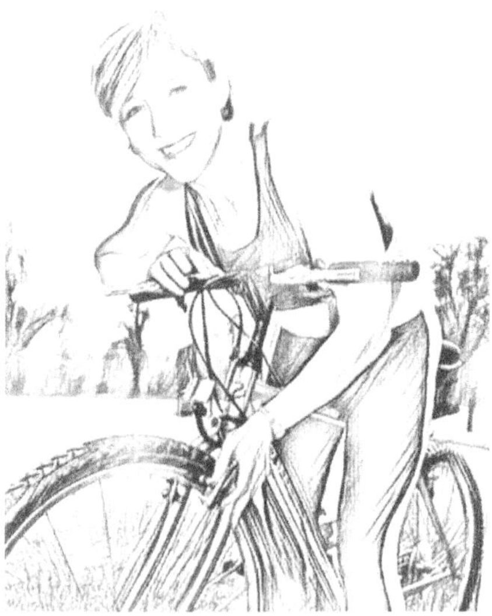

For over a year I had been suffering from very heavy periods and in my job as a physical trainer it was getting very embarrassing. I worked in a gym and ran classes in the park and I trained many clients on a 1-1 basis.

I was 52 years of age and I suspected I was in perimenopause as I was starting to get a little hotter at times, especially at night.

Women can be in this stage of perimenopause for anything between 4 and 10 years and the age at which the first signs start can vary considerably. For some women it can be as young as 30, for others it can start in their mid-40's. It finishes when you have gone 12 months without having a period and then you will have reached your menopause. They say the timing for your menopause is similar, to your mother, but sadly my own mum passed away from cancer when she was just 49 years old so I could not ask her.

I was surprised and embarrassed that I was experiencing this stressful time as I had regular light periods for years and never had Pre-Menstrual Syndrome. (PMS). I rarely had monthly mood changes that many of my friends experienced but now I could empathise with them and their many years of suffering.

At this time, I was teaching spin classes at a health club and I was struggling with very heavy periods and I was worried whether my gym gear would withstand any substantial flow. If you have ever experienced urinary problems, you will know what I mean when the colour of your leggings changes and you get a damp feeling in your pants.
Even writing about it now, I can feel my body heating up the redness developing in my face and the increased heart rate in my chest. Horrible memories!

I really do not know how I continued with teaching and training my clients when I felt so drained and vulnerable. I dreaded my monthly cycle.

Eventually, I was referred to a gynaecologist. He suggested a specific coil to stop the heavy periods, but an internal examination revealed a huge fibroid. This would have to be removed before inserting the coil.
The doctor took a scraping off the lining of the womb at the same time and booked me in for another appointment a week later.
I still remember that appointment as if it were yesterday. My body was used to being in a spin class but on this evening my emotions were thrown into a sudden and mind-numbing spin as my whole life changed.

It was a Thursday evening early 2012 and I was counting the days, looking forward to Saturday 18th February when I was to fly to Kenya and cycle 400 km raising funds for the charity consortium, *Women V Cancer.*

My husband and our best friend were taking me out for dinner as a send-off and I had arranged to meet them at the restaurant just after my follow up appointment.

As I said, I won't forget the *'little chat'* at the hospital that evening. I thought it a little strange that the doctor had 2 nurses with him and they sat at the table and faced me, as an interview situation.

And then I heard him say that I would not be having the coil fitted after all. I heard him say the words I did not want to hear that my womb lining had signs of what he referred to as some 'nasty cells' that had to be removed without delay. I was shocked and speechless. He continued and told me I was booked in for a full hysterectomy in 4 days. At this point, the rest of his words sounded like an echo coming into my head from a place far, far away. The people in front of me faded with blurred edges. Memories of my mum's cancer came back to me and I came out from what seemed like a trance state and anxiously asked the doctor if I had cancer.

His eyes were black and wide as he stared at me, I felt scared as he seriously replied and said he preferred to use the words *'nasty cells'* because they were at an early stage in their development but yes, he had found cancer cells in the lining of my womb that needed to be removed very quickly and all would be well.

At this point my mind spontaneously left the emotions of the situation and went straight into everything I had been planning for the past year. How was I to explain that in two days I was to board a plane to Kenya where I would spend 2 weeks cycling to raise money for 3 well known cancer charities?

It seemed that more than ever I was destined to do this challenge so, I looked at him straight across the table straight into his eyes and asked if we could postpone the operation for just 2 weeks. I explained why and to my joy he agreed. I would arrive home on the Sunday and the operation was booked for the Monday at 10am. It was a tough and emotional cycle ride but it helped me to feel proactive. Not only was I determined to reach my fundraising goal for the charities but I also knew that I was going to do everything I could to beat the cancer.

I am still in touch with many of those wonderful women on that ride many of whom also had their own cancer stories to share. I learned so much from them and I was humbled by their individual perseverance and achievements.

GOODBYE CANCER, HELLO MENOPAUSE

I was 53 years old and the hysterectomy plunged me into menopause and all that goes with it. These were small changes at first. I soon noticed that I would be in T-shirts when others would be in jumpers.

At night, I struggled with my changing body temperature and I would play the game of covers off, covers on, all through the night, after night, after night. My clothes started to get tighter around my middle. One evening, I looked down at my legs and I had never seen them so wide, I honestly believed, that they belonged to someone else. I also had a new wake up time of 3.30am every morning, without an alarm and that was every single morning. Sex became a painful effort as I *'dried up'* and I lost my libido and interest in intimacy. I feared this would be a permanent condition and that it would severely affect my relationship with my husband.

I also, endured the most terrible mood swings and I cried at the most ridiculous things I could not watch TV without constantly welling up with tears. However, when the biggest and cruelest change came it sabotaged my confident, happy personality altogether.

ANXIETY

Like many women I found myself struggling to keep my life and my business going, whilst dealing with my changing daily emotions. I believed everyone was better than me, I believed they were stronger, fitter, prettier, slimmer, and more knowledgeable than me. I questioned my own abilities, even though I had been in the fitness industry for over 20 years.

Overcoming fears that I had not experienced before became a daily battle. I practised deep breathing exercises before my clients arrived, to ward off the cloud of negativity that constantly surrounded me. There were many desperate times when I seriously thought about giving up my business as I no longer felt good enough to continue.

However, I managed to get through an uncertain and unhappy year after the hysterectomy, but I kept searching for help and a solution that would ease my plight. I could not see an end to my experience and had no idea when it would stop.

So, skipping forward a year, I attended a brilliant Women's Health Conference where after an impressive presentation from a speaker on solutions to menopausal symptoms I made the decision to take Bio Identical Hormones.

It was a personal choice and I did not go into it lightly. My GP was amazing and she shared her views with me and regarding the cost, she said, *"It's the cost of a weekend away Julie."* That afternoon I made the appointment at the Marion Gluck Clinic and within a couple of weeks I began Hormone Replacement Therapy (HRT).

It may sound dramatic, but these pills honestly changed my life. I took them for 5 years but after just a few months my husband said, *"It felt great to have my Julie back again"*.

The therapy was not a cheap option at £500.00 (2013) for all the initial blood tests and appointments and then a regular monthly cost of £45 for the plant-based tablets. Many women choose the common types of HRT available on the NHS and I know they have had varying experiences. There are also many women who worry about the links between HRT and Breast Cancer. Please look at the up-to-date research on the NHS website so that you can read for yourself, the latest facts.

However, for me it was a clear decision, because to feel like 'Me' again and to be able to run my business, enjoy my relationship with husband and have my social life back again. Well, it was worth every penny. My personal philosophy is that life is for living but I was not living my life to the full at all for over a year following the hysterectomy and it was frustrating and demoralising.

This therapy gave me my life back. I continued to have a warm and loving relationship with my husband returned to my activities and expanded my business. I was happy again.

Up until that experience I had never thought about how drastically and suddenly, a woman's body changes immediately following surgical menopause. But here I was experiencing the many symptoms I had read about but did not think would be relevant to me personally. I had an awakening and I understood all the many annoying symptoms that so many of my clients had shared with me over the years. Suddenly, I was in the same camp and finally realised how strong my wonderful older friends had been.

Mid Life Crisis, they called it. We all know that you cannot just take a pill and everything will be OK. You have a headache and take paracetamol but you may need to lie down to drink plenty of water and maybe eat something if your sugar levels are low. You get an infection or a virus and need antibiotics but you may need to take time off work to rest to find positive mental attitude to help you recover quicker.

I was on HRT but needed to make lifestyle changes to get the best out of my pill.

I needed to:

- Change my way of exercising.
- Revise my eating habits.
- Lower my alcohol consumption.
- Organise my daily routines and my night-time rituals.
- Look at some serious 'life laundry'.

By the end of this chapter, I want you to feel more in control of a part of your body that you may not feel you can discuss openly and freely.

Many women keep quiet and are secretive about their symptoms, which can be an enormous strain on their emotional and mental health. They keep their secret hidden hoping they will get over it when the menopause finishes. Many women also feel that buying incontinence pads is an easier and less public solution but urinary incontinence, stress incontinence and urinary urgency are life debilitating for a lot of women. Only a small number of women who suffer will speak up and be honest about their own incontinence even though a high ratio of women over the age of 40 have an overactive bladder.

Why should you have to prepare yourself before you can run, jump and play?

Why should you have to worry about sneezing, laughing or coughing?

I am a great believer in changing with the times and I was and still am researching and learning new skills so I can be the best trainer and coach I can be.

In 2013, I trained to be a coach with Burrell Education and specialised in the Holistic Core Restore® programme. One of the many programmes available for women, for all women wherever they may be on life wonderful cycle.

There are 11 offerings and there is a programme for every woman, at every life phase. I feel extremely proud to have an ongoing high level of education from the programme's creator, Jenny Burrell. I feel extremely proud that I have the skills and the empathy to help so many women.

Age is not a factor when it comes to dysfunction, nor is size or health. It can strike at any time and I wanted to learn more so I could help more women. I wanted to make a difference and speak out confidently when talking about our most intimate area It is such an important part of our body and it should not be ignored.

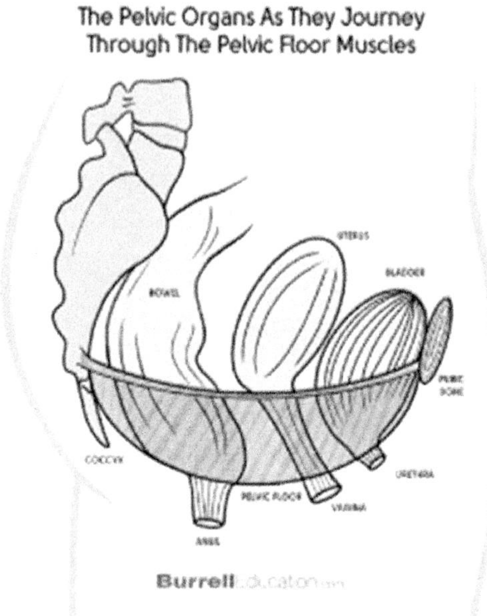

HOW TO CONNECT AND STRENGTHEN YOUR PELVIC FLOOR AND CORE MUSCLES

Firstly, let us start with some basic anatomy. What is your pelvic floor?

Many women will answer and say, *"That's the part that you squeeze to stop you peeing yourself"* but it is so much more than that.

As you can see from the diagram, it is not just about squeezing the vaginal opening closed. Look at the complex anatomy above your openings. Look at how the organs sit above your pelvic floor *'hammock.'* Look at how your pelvic floor muscles connect between the pubic bone and the coccyx.

The first step I take to help my clients strengthen their pelvic floor and core is to start with their breathing.

How do you breathe? Take a moment and look at yourself in the mirror, as you take a deep breath in.

Do your shoulders lift?

Does your chest puff out and your stomach suck in?

Does your rib cage move?

Now take time to relax (seated or standing) and this time take a deep breath in through your nose and bring your awareness to your ribs, front, sides and back. Put your hands there so you can direct your breath into this area. Focus and breathe through your nose with your mouth closed if possible. If you have breathing difficulties or asthma, breathe in a way that suits you but still directing it into the chest and ribs. Feel your lungs expand, your ribs expanding front sides and back without raising your shoulders.

Do this a few times and then rest.

Breathe deeply into your ribs, front, sides and back and then fill your stomach with your breath. Feel it expand. Breathe right down to your pubic bone before breathing out through your mouth.

For many of you this will be hard work because you are probably used to holding your tummy in not expanding it out.

Give yourself time and try it lying on your back with your knees bent. You may find lying down easier. Feel each breath connecting with your stomach.

Closing your eyes can help and placing your hands on your stomach, so that you can feel it rise can also help.

Sometimes this can take a whole session with a client to get this right.

Now breathe out through pursed lips.

Once you feel you have mastered the *'in breath,'* work on your *'out breath'*.

Breathe out through your mouth, a purposeful breath, something you can hear, like a long sigh, but through pursed lips. Think of a steam train coming to a halt and that blast of steam you hear as it stops. Practise this a few times; breathe in through your nose then breathe out through your mouth.

Now let us concentrate on the connection. You have connected with your breath, now you want to connect to the pelvic floor and core muscles, as shown earlier. Once you have started breathing out through pursed lips, you need to connect to the muscles in your vagina, your anus, your lower tummy, your back, your sides, and your diaphragm. Think about drawing your belly button back to your spine as you slowly draw up from your pelvic floor muscles to your diaphragm under your rib cage. Really focus on each body part as you slowly and purposefully breathe out and connect to each point.

Place this book down so you can read and follow the instructions step by step until it becomes a fluid and connecting movement. I am going to use the analogy of a steam train during this exercise. You can do this lying on your back with your knees bent, seated with your feet grounded on the floor or standing with your feet grounded. Do this in bare feet so you can feel the connection between the floor and your feet.

Now, try again but now you are going deeper and now include your stomach.

1. Give yourself a little shake to relax. Shoulders down, rib cage down and plant your feet firmly on the ground. Deep breath in through your nose, filling your ribs, front back and side and fill your tummy all the way down to your pubic bone.

2. Open your mouth slightly and breathe out through pursed lips, (think steam train and lift your core muscles on board that train) As you start to breathe out, switch on to the muscles you use when you pee and the muscles you use if you wanted to stop the passing of wind. Close and lift your vagina and your anus. Practise this a few times, making sure you release everything in-between breaths. Imagine your steam train now has your undercarriage on board.

3. Now that you have connection with your vagina and anus on your 'out breath take your awareness to the muscles a little higher, at your hips. The muscle layer at the front and sides of your abdominal wall is called the Transverse Abdominal Muscle, the TVA. This muscle is nicknamed the '*corset muscle'* and rightly so, as I have had many clients report a flatter tummy simply by engaging these muscles on a regular basis with the exercises I give them, known which I call '*tummy vacuums.* I will share this exercise with you later as your TVA muscles are vital to your core and back strength and are your body's natural belt.

4. So, get them on board the steam train. Now, you have drawn up your vagina and your anus muscles, on your *'out breath'* and now, your awareness is on your TVA muscles. Imagine pulling those muscles into the centre to your belly button and into your spine.

5. Keep this tension below your belly button for now. Keep practicing, to feel a deep connection between your pelvic floor muscles and your transverse abdominal muscles.

6. So, now you have your vaginal muscles, your anus, and your transverse abdominal muscles on board. Now to include your back into the exercise; think of pulling your pubic bone and your coccyx (tailbone) together. Still breathing out through pursed lips, connect and draw these muscles up and onto the 'train.' It sometimes helps to place your hands on your

tummy and feel the muscles move away from your hands. Breathe out, connect, and draw up and in. You can also place a hand on your coccyx and you should feel the muscles tighten as you connect here.

7. All aboard, well nearly. Now, continue further up your body and draw your sides (oblique muscles) in and up towards your diaphragm, just under your ribs. Your diaphragm is the major muscle of respiration. As you breathe in this muscle flattens and presses down, sucking air into your lungs. As you breathe out, your diaphragm relaxes and air is forced out of your lungs.

I like to think of it as an umbrella due to its shape in the lower part of the rib cage. When I breathe out deeply, my diaphragm relaxes upwards, pulling everything up with it and when I connect to my pelvic floor muscles, I can feel my whole core area strengthen.

Now, put all the above together and you have the first step towards connecting and strengthening your pelvic floor.

It takes time and commitment. I spend 6 sessions working with people with pelvic floor dysfunction but from the feedback I have had in the past it is worth every minute. Not worrying about whether you should jump and not worrying about crossing your legs when you sneeze especially not worrying about wearing pads every day is a blessing that every woman should experience.

I believe you cannot strengthen what you cannot connect to. So, spend time on feeling the connection between breathing out and the contraction of your pelvic floor and core muscles and you will feel the benefit very quickly. Clients have reported better orgasms, less leakage, less urgency, and more confidence.

This is just the beginning of your road to a fully functional pelvic floor and core. The next step is to add in resistance and movement. I would love to hear from you and help you on your journey to a life full of joy and confidence.

These simple exercises will work. You need to do the work and YOU will get the results.

Here are some of the testimonials I have received since delivering the programme.

"Julie has given me the confidence and strength to heal physically and mentally."

"I have more bladder control and I feel fitter and firmer."

"I really enjoyed the course and the positive support Julie gives. I feel I have so much more control now."

"I can walk the children to school now without worrying about peeing myself."

"Worth every penny, I have my body back and it is thanks to Julie Bartlett and her magic."

This inspiring quote sums up why my clients get so much out of working with me.

> *"I've learned that people will forget what you said.*
> *People will forget what you did. But people will*
> *never forget how you made them feel."*

Maya Angelou

Activist, Poet, Author, Singer and Actress

I know my clients feel so much better, confident, and empowered. This is just the beginning of what the Holistic Core Program® is all about and I am pleased to able to deliver this both 1-1 and online. Please visit my website for full details.

Julie Bartlett is a double award-winning Personal Trainer who specialises in helping women overcome the unhappiness of pelvic floor dysfunction and prolapse She overcame many health issues herself and now enjoys empowering others. **www.juliebartlett.me**

Appreciation

Thank you Sarah, Alison and Julie for contributing your professional expertise to this book. I believe that women should work together to make this world a better place for everyone and I deeply, believe that the true power that women hold, is in their natural ability to intuitively, support and nurture each other.

Thank you ladies, you are incredible.

~ Pause Here ~

Dear Reader

I trust that you have found this book useful and that you will use the techniques and the information to question your beliefs about ageing and its effects on your self-perception and what is possible for you in your future.

My Sincerest Wish For You

is that you
wake up every morning with energy and confidence,
loving what you see in your mirror,
feeling ready to have a great day and
enjoying 'being YOU again'.

Victoria

♡

References

Age U.K., (2017), Money and Mental Health Policy Institute, *Seeing through the Fog*, www.ageuk.org.uk

BBC, (2021), U.K. *Physical, emotional and social wellbeing* - Health and wellbeing - WJEC - GCSE Physical Education Revision - WJEC - BBC Bitesize. UK

Flegal, K. Dr. et al, (2013), Association of All-Cause Mortality With Overweight and Obesity Using Standard Body Mass Index Categories". *JAMA*. **309** (1): 71-28. doi: 10.1001/jama. 012.113905. PMC 4855514. PMID 23280227 USA

Frostrup, M., Smellie A., (2022), Cracking The Menopause: While Keeping Yourself Together, Revised version, Bluebird, London, UK

Grabowska, W. Sikora, E and Bielak-Zmiiewska, A. (2017), Sirtuins, A Promising Target in Slowing Down the Ageing Process 10.1007/s10522-017-9685-9 https://www.ncbi.nlm.nih.gov/pmc/articles/PMC5514220/

Hannon, K. (2019), *Never too old to Get Rich: The Entrepreneur's Guide to Starting a Business Mid-Life,* John Wiley & Sons, New Jersey, USA.

Hay, L. (1984), *You Can Heal Your Life,* Hay House, London, UK

Hicklin, T. Ph.D., (2016), https://www.nih.gov/news-events/nih-research-matters/molecular-ties-between-lack-sleep-weight-gain U.S.A.

Iliff, J. Ph.D. and Nedergaard, M. Ph.D., University of Rochester, Medical Center, (2012), New York, USA https://www.nih.gov/news-events/nih-research-matters/how-sleep-clears-brain USA

Jerath, R. et al, (2006), *Physiology of long pranayamic breathing:* Neural respiratory elements may provide a mechanism that explains how slow deep breathing shifts the autonomic nervous system, Medical Hypothesis, 67, 566-571. USA

Keller, H. et al, (1991), *The Story of My Life,* Bantam Classic, New York, U.S.A

Luders, E. et al, (2015), *Forever Young(er): potential age-defying effects of long-term meditation on gray matter atrophy,* Department of Neurology, School of Medicine, University of California, Los Angeles, Los Angeles, CA, USA. https://www.sciencedaily.com

Maslow, A.H. (2013), *Theory of Human Motivation,* Martino Publishing Mansfield Centre, CT, USA

Mitteldorf, D. Dr. and Sagan, C. Dr. (2017), Cracking The Ageing Code: The New Science of Growing old – And What It Means For Staying Young, Flatiron Books, USA

Morhenn, V. Beavin. L. and Zak. P, *Massage Increases Oxytocin and Reduces Adrenocorticotroin Hormone in Humans*, (2012), University of California, USA

Mott, M. Ph.D., (2021), UK. https://www.nih.gov/news-events/nih-research-matters/brain-protein-affects-aging-sleep

National Health Service, (2019), UK. https://www.nhs.uk/live-well/sleep-and-tiredness/how-to-get-to-sleep

Newson, L Dr and Lewis. R, Dr (2022), https://www.newsonhealth.co.uk/new-patient-faqs

Northrup, C. (2015), *Goddesses Never Age*, Hay House, London, UK

Pal, G.K. Velkumary, S. and Madanmohan, (2015), *Effect of short-term practice of breathing exercises on autonomic functions:* in normal human volunteers. Indian Journal of Medical Research, India

Reumel, M. (2022), *Tips for Mature Women* https://www.youtube.com/watch?v=NeHp_blzVB8

Stoyanov, S. Ph.D., (2017), *Abraham H Maslow's; A theory of Human Motivation,* Macat Library; 1st edition Scotland UK

Websites

https://www.**ageuk**.org.uk/ 2022
https://blog.**biosearchtech**.com/buddy-up-the-double-helix/ 2016
https://www.**burrelleducation**.co.uk/ 2022
https://www.**gov.uk/**government/publications/application-for-a-state-pension-statement/ 2022
https://www.**gov.uk**/individual-savings-accounts/ 2022
https://www.**gov.uk/**power-of-attorney/ 2022
https://www.**mindyourreality**.com/ 2022
https://www.**moneyandmentalhealth**.org/ 2022
https://www.**ncbi**.nlm.gov/pmc/articles/ 2022
https://www.**newsonhealth**.co.uk/ 2022
https://www.**nhs.uk/**live-well/sleep-and-tiredness/ 2022
https://www.**pensionwise**.gov.uk/en/ 2022
https://www.**youtube**.com/watch?v=NeHp_blzVB8 2022

Images

Affirmations

Rejuvenate Your Life

Victoria Sheridan

If you would like to know more
because you want more in your *'Seenager'* years
you can contact me at
www.victoriasheridancoach.com
or email me here
victoria@victoriasheridancoach.com

the Secret Calm

Published by
The Secret Calm Ltd,
Kent, England UK

Printed in Great Britain
by Amazon

82119279R00132